Brace Yourself

Everything You Need to Know About AFOs After Stroke

Jennifaye V. Brown

PT, MSPT, PhD, NCS, CAPS

Copyright © 2024 Jennifaye V. Brown. All rights reserved.

No part of this publication may be reproduced, stored in a retrieval system or transmitted in any form or by any means, electronic, digital, mechanical, photo-copying, photographic, recording, nor may it otherwise be reproduced for private or public use without the prior written permission of the author. For information about permission, please contact the author at info@jvbneuropt.com.

Submit inquiries for author speaking engagements and bulk book print orders to info@jvbneuropt.com.

Photography: Gavin Gilbert Shelton and Jennifaye V. Brown (unless otherwise credited)

Cover Design: Chris Boyer

Printed in the United States of America

ISBN: 979-8-89705-847-1 (Softcover)

ISBN: 979-8-89705-848-8 (e-Book)

Dedication

To my parents Russell E. Brown, Sr. and Mary Louise Steplight Brown who taught me by what they said and did not say and their actions of love the best way they knew how in the moment.

To all of the individuals with stroke whom I served as their physical therapist and allowed me to help them put their best foot forward in an AFO (leg and foot brace)…I am grateful for the opportunity to have learned from you and perfect my craft of designing AFOs.

Table of Contents

Preface - My Foot Journey 6

Introduction 8

Chapter 1 - Definitions and Pictures 9

Chapter 2 - What Is Foot Drop? 24

Chapter 3 - What Is An AFO? 32

Chapter 4 - Why Do I Need An AFO? 34

Chapter 5 - What Should My PT Do? 36

Chapter 6 - What Should I Ask My PT? 39

Chapter 7 - What Should My Orthotist Do? 41

Chapter 8 - What Should I Ask My Orthotist? 43

Chapter 9 - What To Expect When I Get the AFO: Fit & Function 47

Chapter 10 - Physical Therapy Pearls From Career Experiences 50

Afterward 52

References 53

Publications 57

Peer Reviewed Scientific and Professional Presentations 58

About the Author 59

PREFACE

My Foot Journey

At a very young age, I was blessed with long narrow flat feet. My shoe size peeked at a size 12 4A (extremely narrow) and it was very difficult for me to find shoes that fit properly for the activity of school, sports, and formal occasions such as church, graduations, and sorority events. Finding the right shoe for fit and function became my passion when treating individuals with stroke, particularly women who required a foot brace (AFO: ankle foot orthosis).

   I was put to the test when an Atlanta socialite told me she does not own a pair of tennis shoes. And thus, my journey began to create a better AFO to accommodate shoes regularly worn by people. Also, I wanted to design an AFO that addresses specific foot and leg problems instead of ordering a standard AFO as I was taught at the University of Miami (FL) Physical Therapy Program. I decided to apply what I know about the human body, particularly the leg and foot from a neurological (brain and nerves) and musculoskeletal (muscles and bones) point of view and take into consideration activities from sit to stand to walking and running to make the best custom AFO. I focus on a person's lifestyle from daily activities to the type of clothes and shoes worn during those activities. Using my creative spirit to develop therapy exercises and activities based on social determinants of health[1] (education access and quality, economic stability, health care access and quality, neighborhood and built environment, and social and community context [people]), I design distinct types of AFOs which can be later made by an orthotist. I have conducted research regarding how people feel about their AFOs and physical therapists' knowledge and use of specific tests to assess them for fit and function and whether test information is used to justify reimbursement from the insurance company. I have published articles about my findings.

Through the years, I have designed an assortment of AFOs and learned some valuable lessons along the way. I am excited about sharing the knowledge gained from Emory University - Bachelor of Arts in Psychology, the University of Miami (FL) - Master of Science in Physical Therapy, and the University of South Carolina - Doctor of Philosophy in Exercise Science and pearls of wisdom as a result of working with individuals who have had a brain injury, particularly stroke, and their caregivers.

Introduction

As an individual living with problems as a result of a stroke, you deserve to be the best you. That means looking the way you want and feeling good about yourself to live the life you want. So many of the people I have treated for stroke and other neurologic diagnoses, have shared one thing in common. For many reasons, they did not like the AFO supposedly made to help them walk. Wearing the AFO was more than about walking. It created an identity of who they did not want to be, a person who is not normal and certainly did not look normal. The AFO represented who they were in the moment and would be in the future. I wanted each individual and their caregivers to know that the AFO represented the potential to become an engaged person in life with opportunities that stemmed from the simple act of walking for their health. I had to instill in everyone, including my fellow physical therapy practitioners and orthotists, that we need to make a person-centered AFO that would bring out the best potential of each person to become comfortable and vibrant in him or herself as they lived with the effects of a stroke. A better fitting and looking AFO that reflects the personality of the person in terms of style and function would assure a better health outcome in all dimensions of wellness: mental, physical, psychosocial, spiritual, environmental, and vocational.

I wrote this book particularly for individuals with stroke, their caregivers, physical therapy practitioners, and orthotists. It is a resource that will guide the making of an AFO that a person would want to wear. I hope and believe that it will help anyone with a neurological problem and those who provide care for those individuals.

CHAPTER 1

Definitions and Pictures

The Leg has 2 Bones and 3 Major Structures[2]

- **Tibia:** Wide bone of the inner leg
- **Fibula:** Thin lateral bone of the outer leg
- **Malleoli:** Protruding parts of the tibia and fibula bones on the inside and outside of the ankle
- **Tibial Tuberosity:** Protruding part of the tibia bone below the knee joint

Anterior (Front) View of the Left Leg

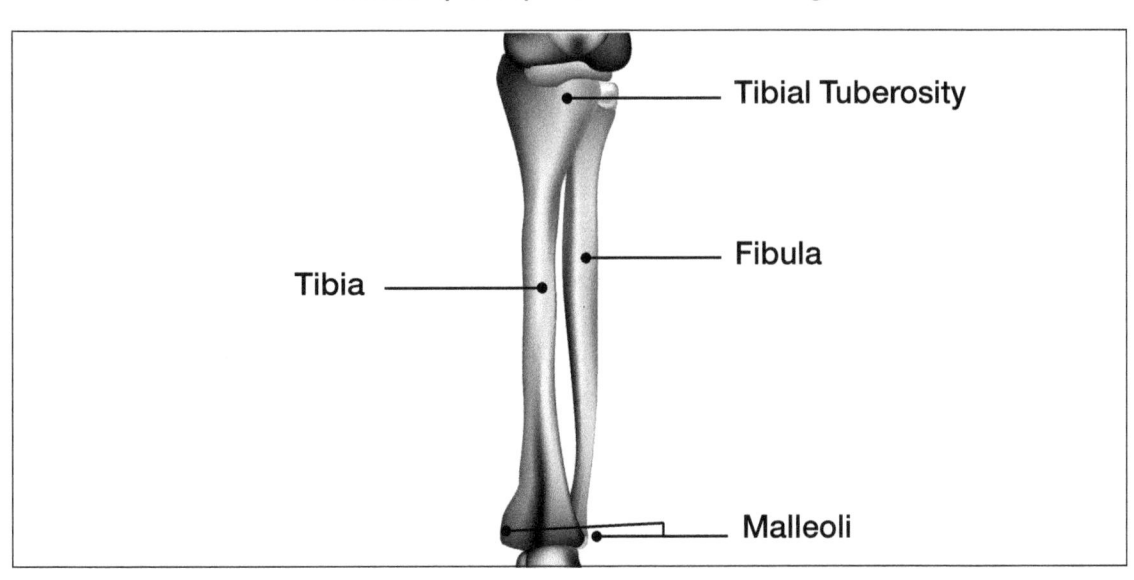

The Foot is Divided into 3 Sections[3-4]

- **Hindfoot:** The calcaneus (heel) and the talus bones
- **Midfoot:** The navicular, cuboid, and cuneiform bones that are connected to the metatarsals (long bones of the foot)
- **Forefoot:** Metatarsals and the phalanges (toes)

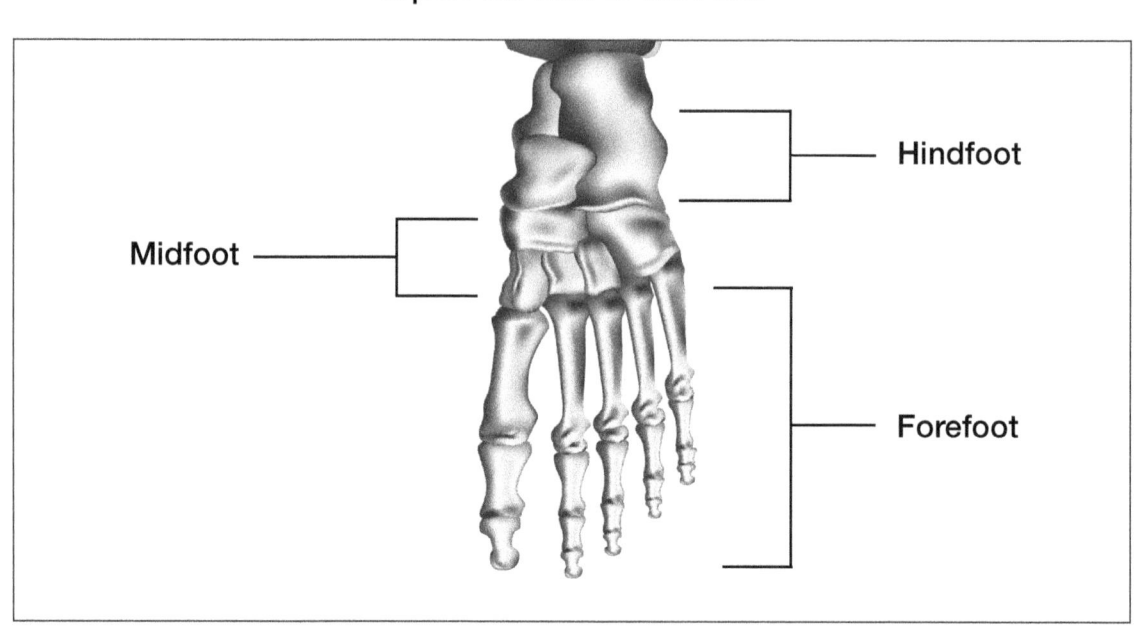

Top Down View of the Foot

The Foot has 26 Bones (major ones listed)[3-4]

- **Calcaneus:** Heel bone
- **Talus:** Bone on top of calcaneus and under the tibia and fibula
- **Navicular:** Inner bone of the midfoot
- **Cuboid:** Outer bone of the midfoot
- **Cuneiforms:** Outer, middle, and inner bones between the navicular and cuboid

- **Metatarsals:** Five long bones of the forefoot whose distal ends are known as metatarsal heads and are connected to the toe bones
- **Phalanges:** The forefoot bones that make up the toes; the big toe has two and the rest of the toes have three

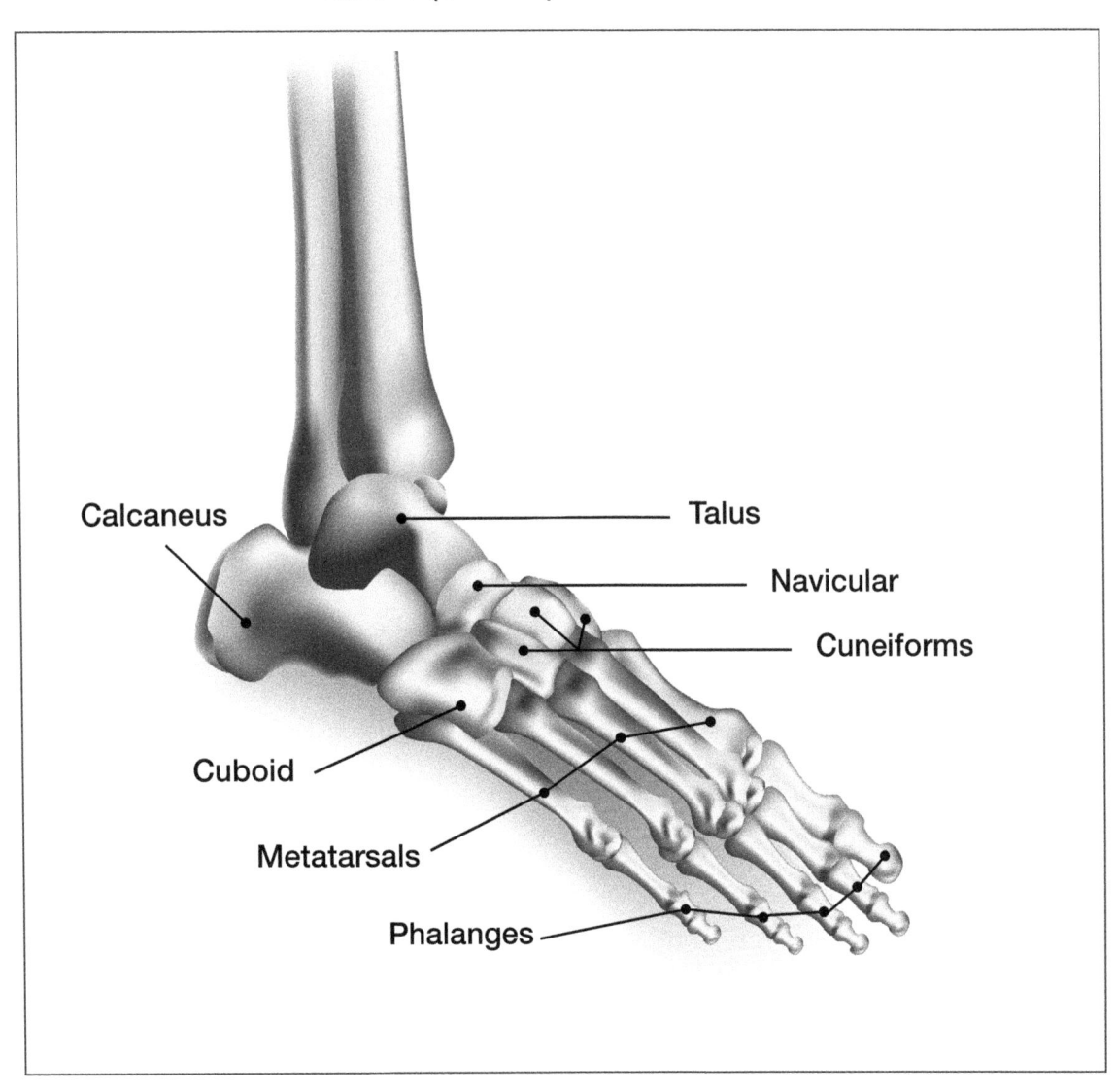

Lateral (Outside) View of the Foot

The Foot is Divided into 3 Arches[3-4]

- **Anterior Transverse Arch:** From base of the big toe to the base of the little toe
- **Medial Longitudinal Arch:** From inside of the heel bone (calcaneus) to the base of the big toe, second, and third toe
- **Lateral Longitudinal Arch:** From outside of the heel bone to the base of the little toe

Lateral (Outside) View of Foot

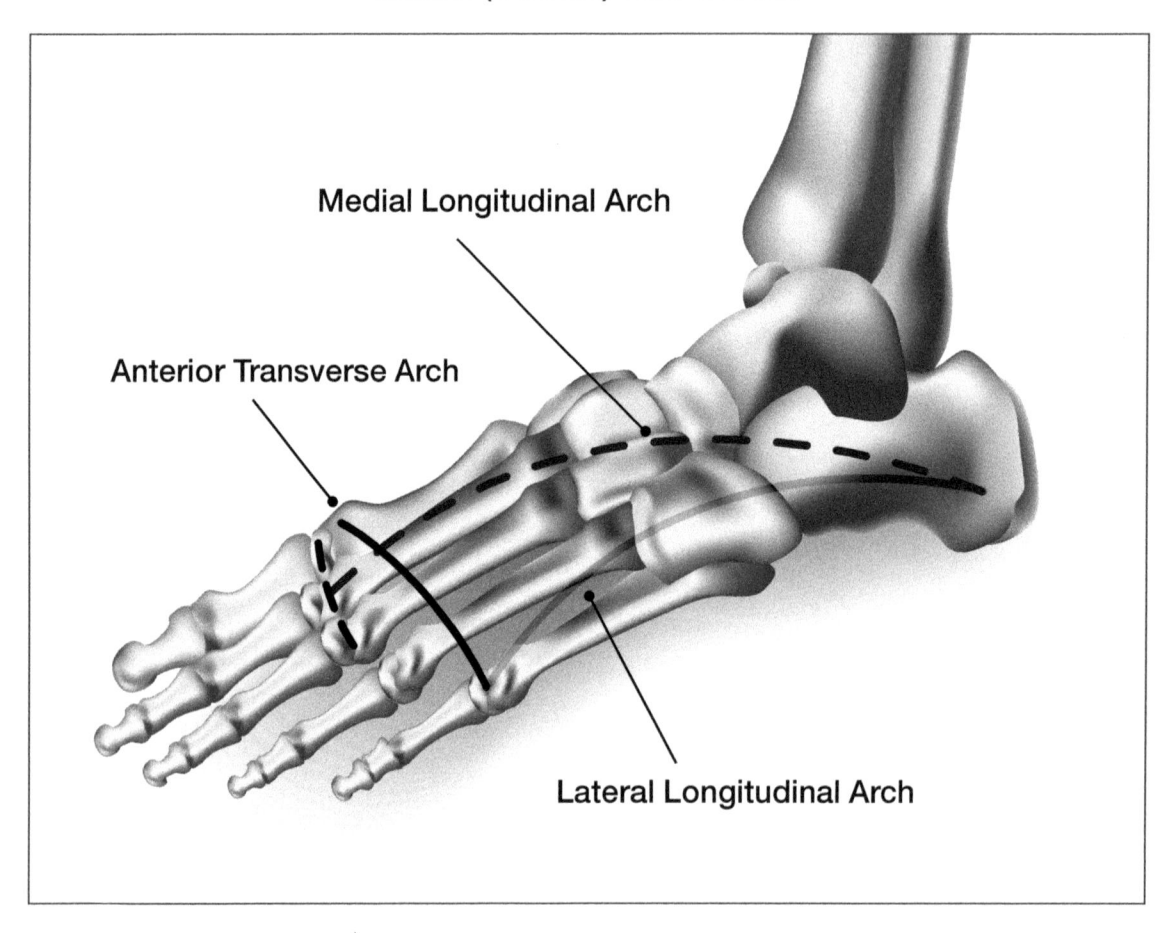

Ankle Foot Orthosis[5] (AFO): A brace for the leg and foot that supports the foot and ankle with the intention to prevent the foot from dragging; it has four major components: posterior calf support connected to a vertical shaft, foot support, closure to secure the brace to the leg and foot (Velstretch®), and five areas of trimlines (edges of the AFO): proximal (top), anterior (front), ankle, foot, and metatarsal (around forefoot)

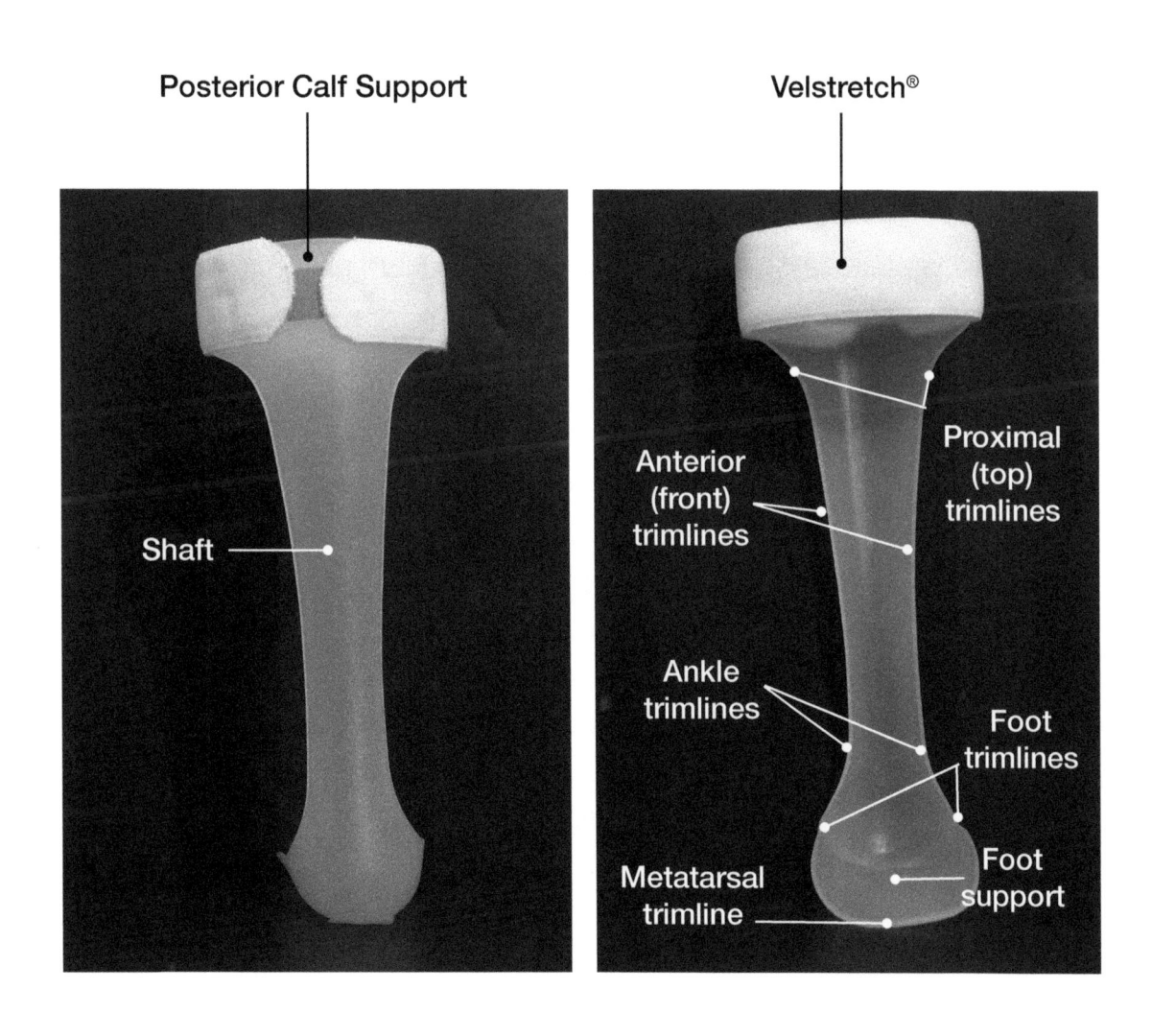

Balance[6]: The ability to maintain center of mass (trunk) over the base of support (feet or hands) by moving the ankles, hips, and or placement of the feet and or hands

Foot Positions[3]

- **Dorsiflexion:** Foot pointed up or when the foot is on a surface, the leg is positioned forward
- **Plantarflexion:** Foot pointed down or when the foot is on a surface, the leg is positioned backward
- **Inversion:** Foot rotated in
- **Eversion:** Foot rotated out
- **Adduction:** Foot movement towards the center of the body
- **Abduction:** Foot movement away from the center of the body

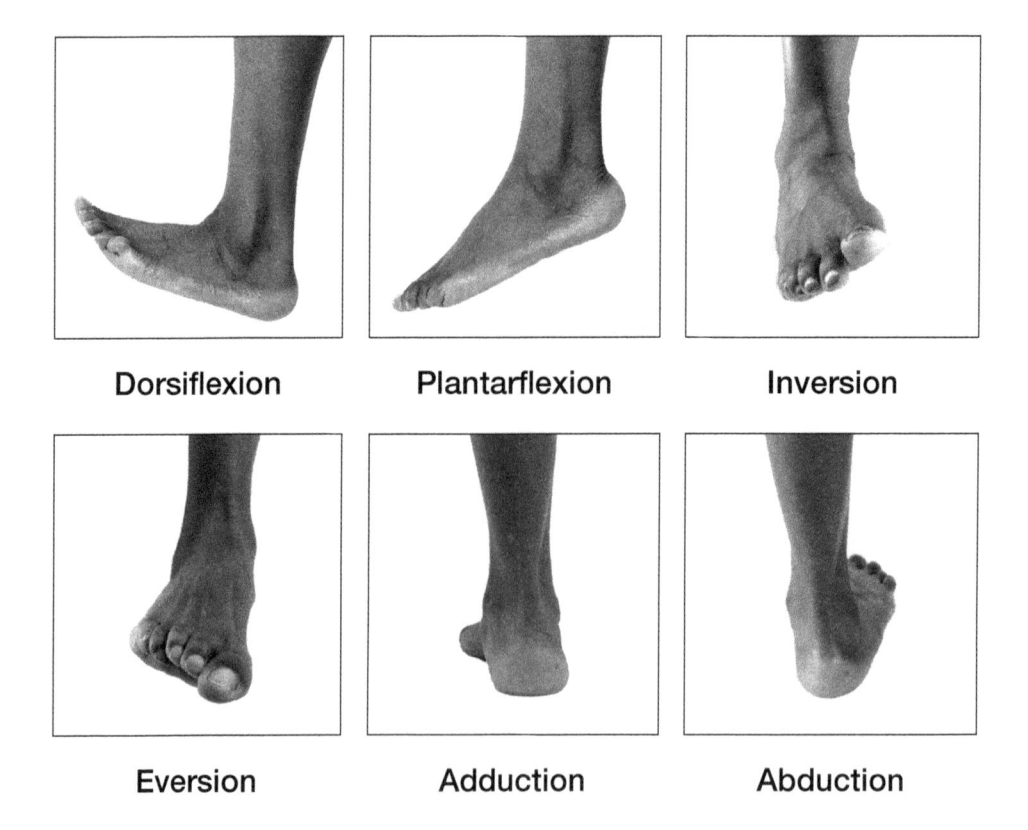

Dorsiflexion   Plantarflexion   Inversion

Eversion   Adduction   Abduction

Foot Appearance[4]

- **Pronation:** Flat foot; the arches of the foot flatten out
- **Supination:** The arch of the inner foot (medial longitudinal arch) is abnormally high

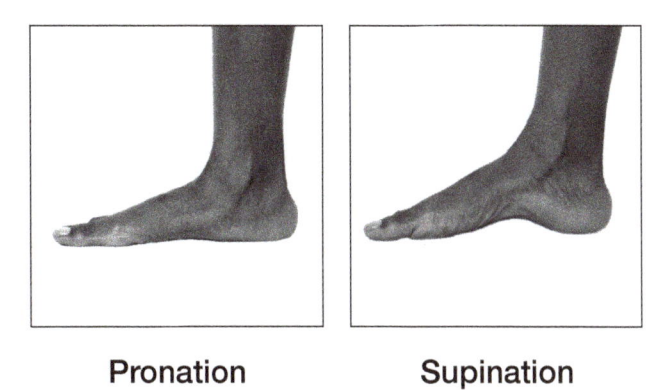

Pronation   Supination

Walking[7-9]: Rhythmical and repetitive movement of the trunk, arm, and leg that requires the act of putting one foot in front of the other to move the body forward; both feet are never off the ground at the same time

Walking Phases[7-9]

- **Swing:** Period of time the foot is off the floor, ground or any surface
- **Stance:** Period of time the foot is on the floor, ground or any surface and body weight moves from behind, over, and in front of the foot

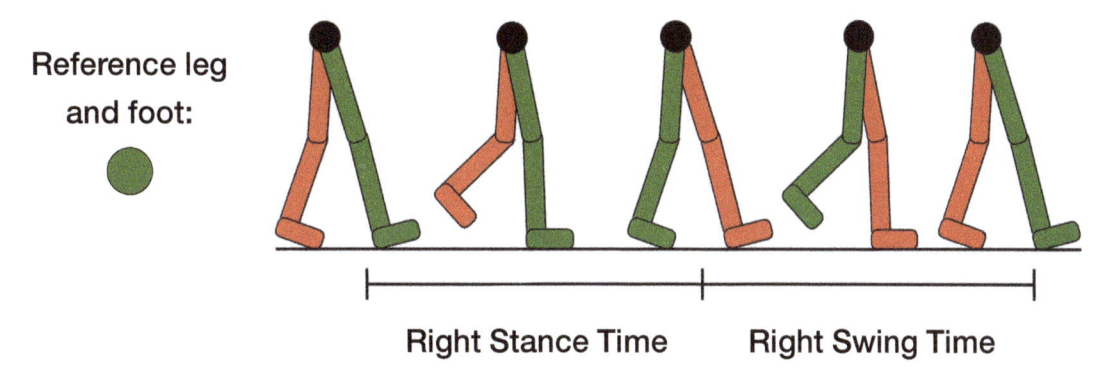

Reference leg and foot:

Right Stance Time   Right Swing Time

Source: Rlawson9, CC BY-SA 3.0 https://commons.wikimedia.org/wiki/File:Gait_Cycle.png

Kinesthesia[10]: Being aware of the amount, speed, and direction of movement

Monofilament testing[10]: A thin plastic wire used to test sensation of the feet

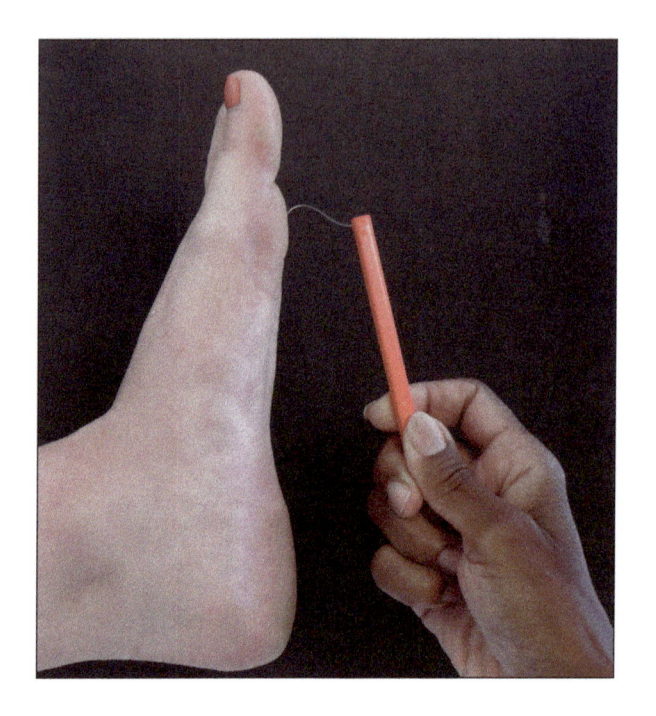

Musculoskeletal[11]: About muscles and bones

Neuromuscular[12]: About the brain, nerves, and muscles

Non-weightbearing[13-14]: The foot is not touching the floor, ground or any surface; the foot is in the air during swing phase of walking

Weightbearing[13-14]: The foot is touching the floor, ground or any surface; load (body weight) is exerted towards the foot causing compression at the joints; the foot is on the floor, ground or any surface during stance phase of walking

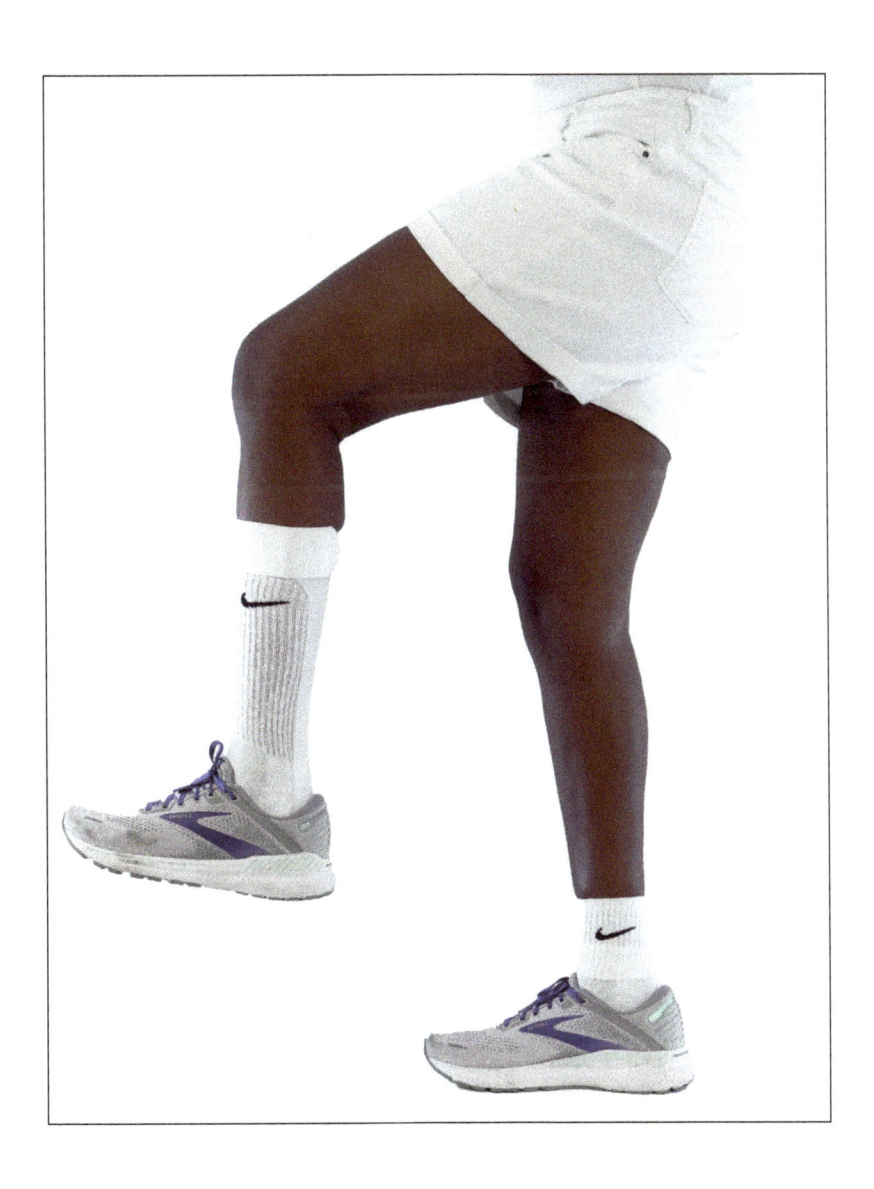

Pathological Reflexes[15]: Abnormal foot movements caused by stimulation to the bottom of the foot; if the reflexes persist, muscles shorten in the direction of foot movement; four pathological reflex movements are toe grasping (bending of the toes), foot movement up, foot rotated in, and foot rotated out

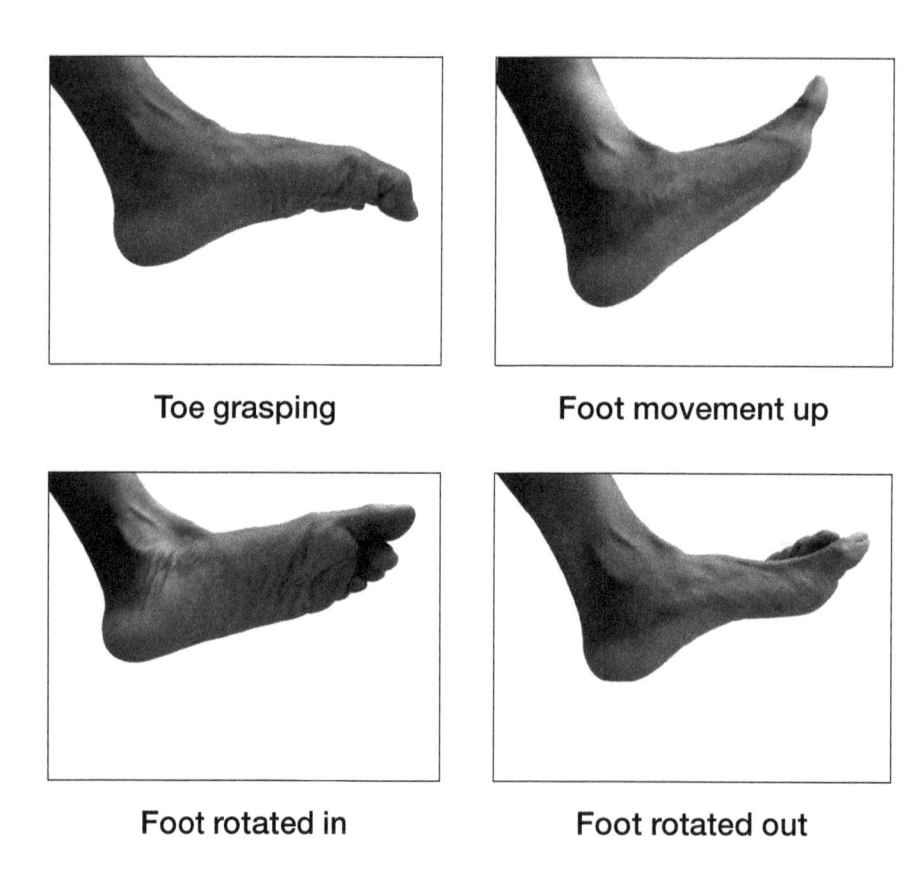

Toe grasping

Foot movement up

Foot rotated in

Foot rotated out

Proprioception[10]: Being aware of a joint (where the end of two bones meet) position

Range of Motion[16]: The amount of movement at a joint which depends on the structures of the joint and flexibility of the muscles that cross the joint; active range of motion is the amount of movement generated by the person and passive range of motion is the amount of movement generated by an external force (for example, a physical therapy practitioner pushing on the foot to measure ankle joint movement)

Recovery[17-18]

- **Functional:** Improvement in the performance of activities, such as sit to stand or walking without necessary improvement in motor function
- **Motor:** Improvement in strength, range of motion, speed, and accuracy of movement in the trunk, upper extremities (shoulder to hand), and or lower extremities (hip to foot)

Shoe Components[19-20]

- **Outsoles:** Bottom layer on the outside of the shoe which comes in contact with the floor, ground or any surface; shoes can have a midsole that can be:

    a. Flat: Causing the shoe to be the same height from the heel to the toes

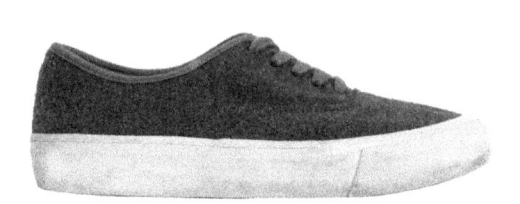

    b. Wedge: Causing the shoe to be higher at the heel and lower at the toes

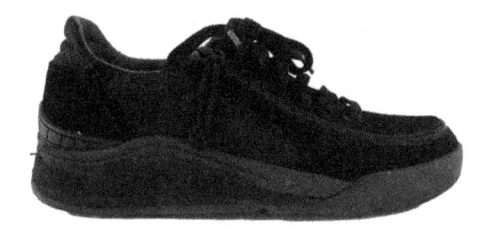

c. Insole: Inside bottom portion which foot is placed; it goes on top of white layer seen in image of shoe below

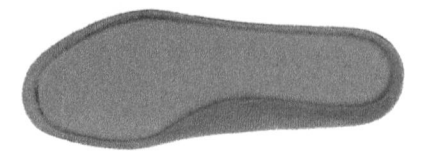

d. Toe box: Area where toes are and can be rounded or pointed

e. Toe cap: Material reinforcement to protect toes at top of the toe box and goes to the sole

f. Vamp: Middle part of the shoe that covers the midfoot and attaches to the flap that covers the top of the foot

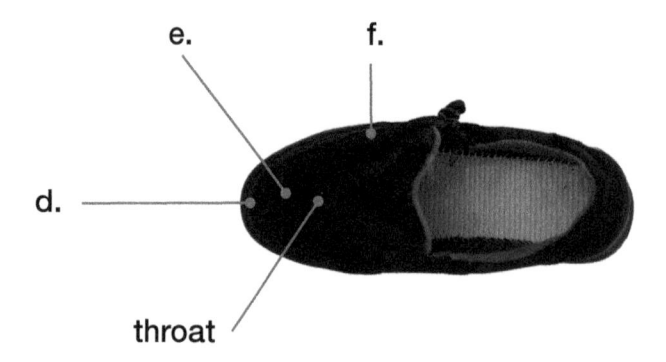

e.
f.
d.
throat

NOTE: The throat is the portion of the flap that attaches to the vamp, and it can be squared or pointed in a shoe.

g. **Quarter:** Portion of the shoe behind vamp and in front of the heel counter or cap

h. **Heel Counter or Cap:** Back part of the shoe that wraps around the heel

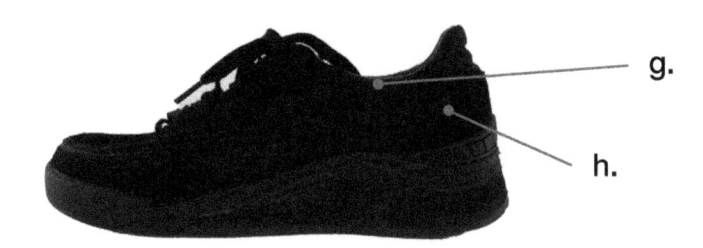

Spasticity[14,21]: A result of damage to motor nerves from the brain when a muscle is stretched at a certain speed; the stretch causes an abnormal reflex response called a clasp-knife like phenomenon; the muscle movement causes the distal body part to look like a clasp-knife closing

Strength[22-23]: A muscle generates force to overcome resistance during a specific circumstance resulting in movement

Abnormal Synergy Patterns[12,21]: Synergy means muscles moving as a group

- **Extension:** Due to damage in the brain, muscles contract in a manner causing the knee to be straight and the foot is pointed down or down and rotated in

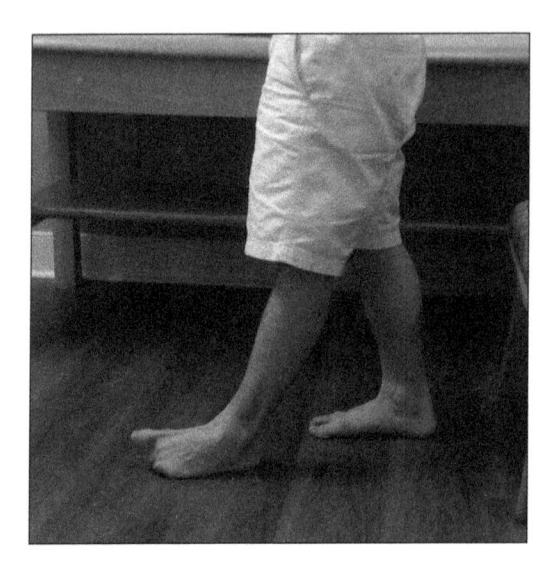

- **Flexion:** Due to damage in the brain, muscles contract in a manner causing the hip and knee to bend and the foot is pointed up and rotated in

Tone[13-14,24]: Muscle tension felt when moving a body part such that a muscle goes from a shortened to a longer position; muscle tone ranges from flaccid (floppy) to low tone to high tone (stiff) or rigid (muscle unable to shorten or lengthen) due to damage of a upper motor neuron in the brain and spinal cord or a lower motor nerve that goes to a muscle

Vision

- **Hemianopsia**[25-26] **(Visual Field Cut):** Brain damage causes the person to see half of everything from each eye
- **Visual Neglect**[25-27]: Damage to parts of the brain that controls vision, sensation, and or movement processing areas; the person is unable to process and interact with what is seen

Paris as Seen with Left Homonymous Hemianopsia

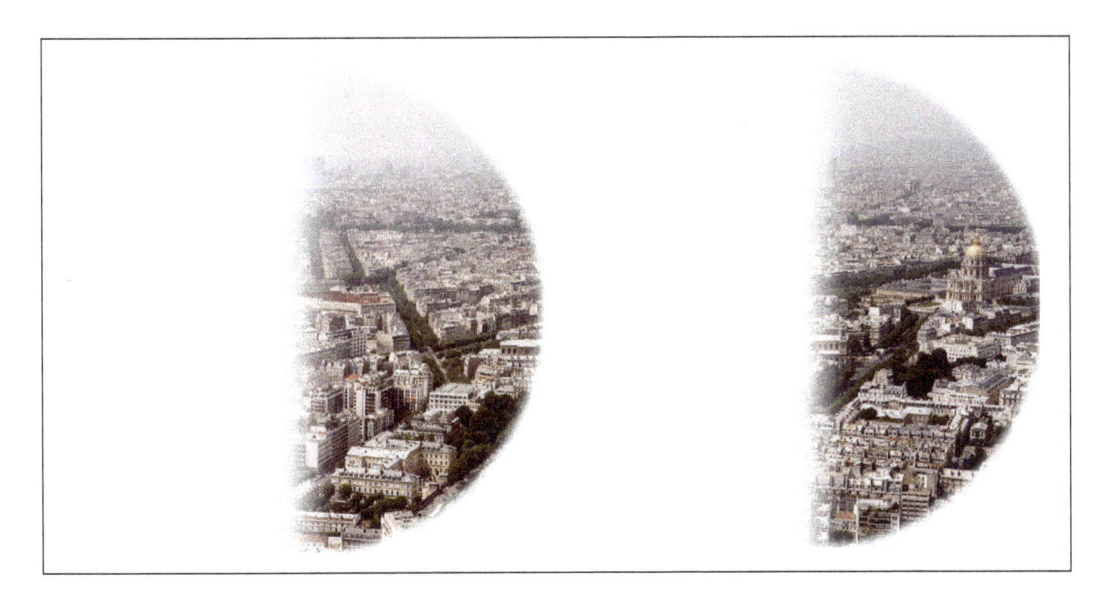

Source: https://commons.wikimedia.org/wiki/File:Paris_as_seen_with_left_homonymous_hemianopsia.png

CHAPTER 2

What Is Foot Drop?

The brain uses neurons (nerve cells that make up the nervous system in the brain and spinal cord) to communicate with different parts of the body. There is an upper motor neuron that leaves the brain and connects with a neuron in the spinal cord which then communicates with a lower motor nerve (a group of nerve cells whose tails are bundled together to form an axon) that leaves the spine and goes to the muscle.

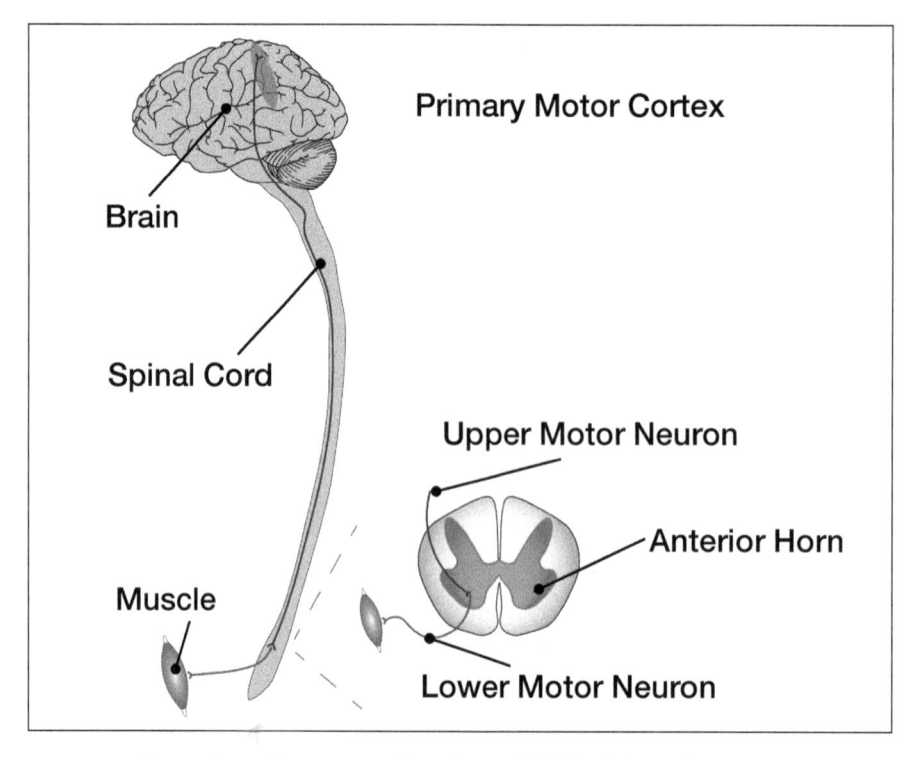

Source: https://commons.wikimedia.org/wiki/File:UMN_vs_LMN.png

The foot is dropped for two reasons:

First, there is damage to the upper motor neuron (corticospinal tract) from the brain that communicates with the lower motor nerve (deep peroneal nerve) that controls the tibialis anterior muscle which pulls the foot up (dorsiflexion) and rotates it in (inversion).

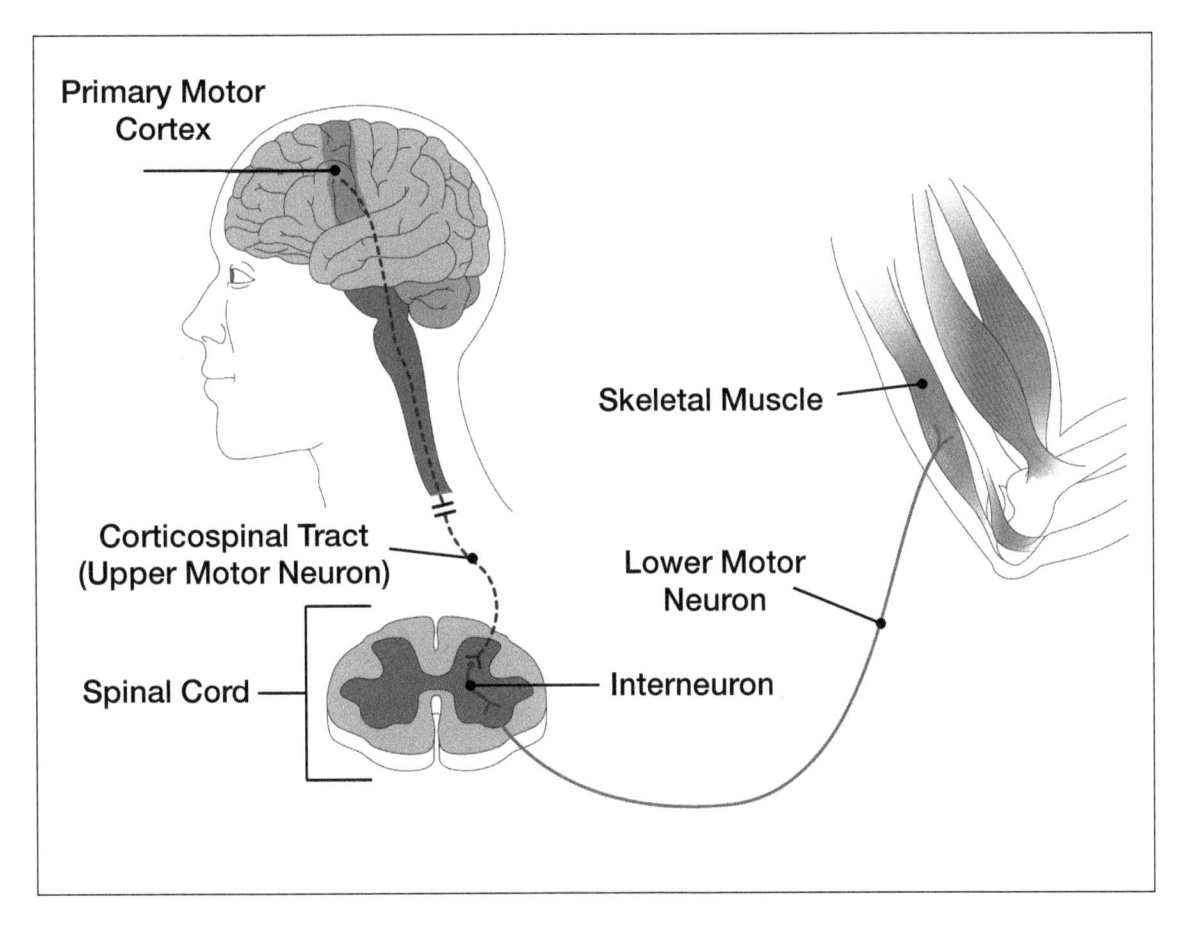

Source: https://commons.wikimedia.org/wiki/File:Illustration_of_the_motor_neuron_tract_descending_from_primary_motor_cortex,_via_spinal_cord,_to_skeletal_muscle.jpg

Anterior (Front) View of Tibialis Anterior

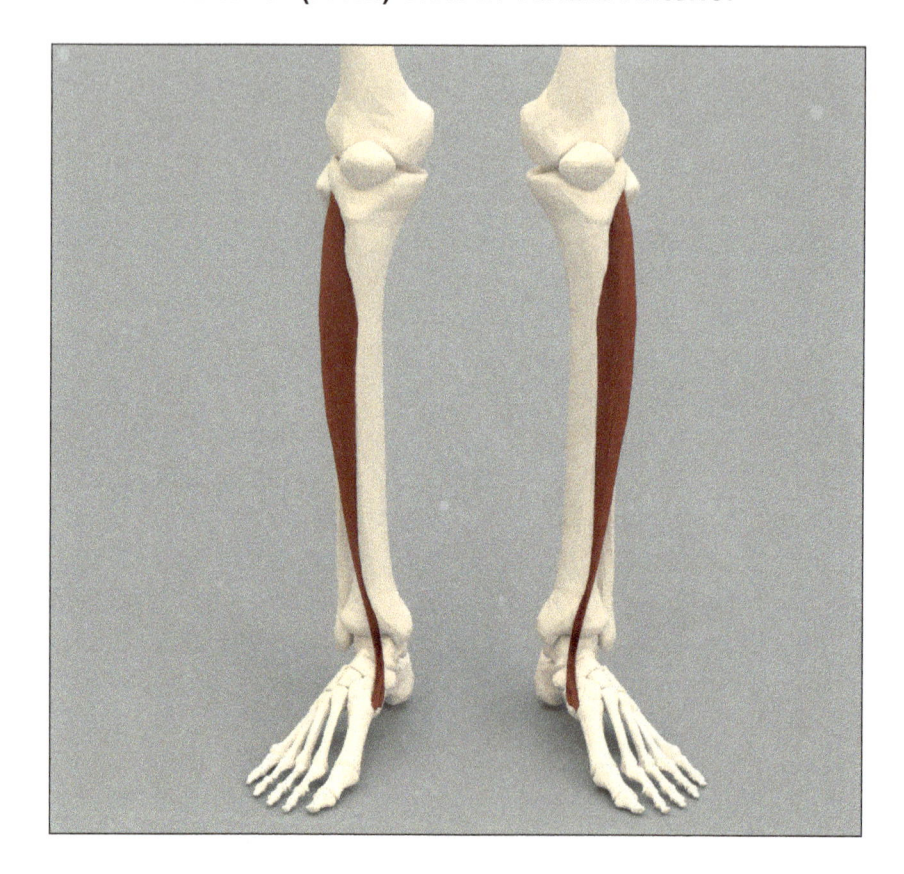

Source: https://commons.wikimedia.org/wiki/File:Tibialis_anterior_muscle_-_anteriror_view.png

There is another muscle that pulls the foot up and rotates it out (eversion) which is called fibularis longus; however, the primary muscle to pull the foot up is the tibialis anterior.

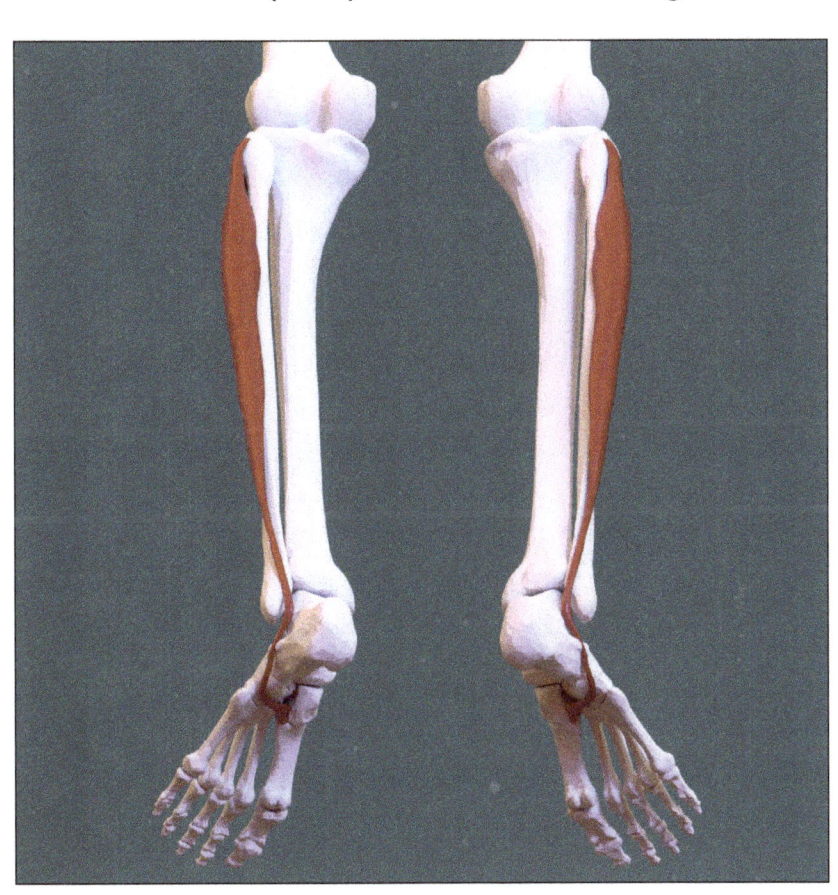

Posterior (Back) View of Fibularis Longus

Source: https://commons.wikimedia.org/wiki/File:Lateral_compartment_of_leg_-_Fibularis_longus.png

In this first example, the foot position tends to be floppy but can become stiff over time.

Second, the upper motor neuron (corticospinal tract) is completely destroyed and unable to communicate with other upper motor neurons. These other upper motor neurons cause the knee to be straight and the foot to point down (plantar-flexion) or down and rotated in (equinovarus).

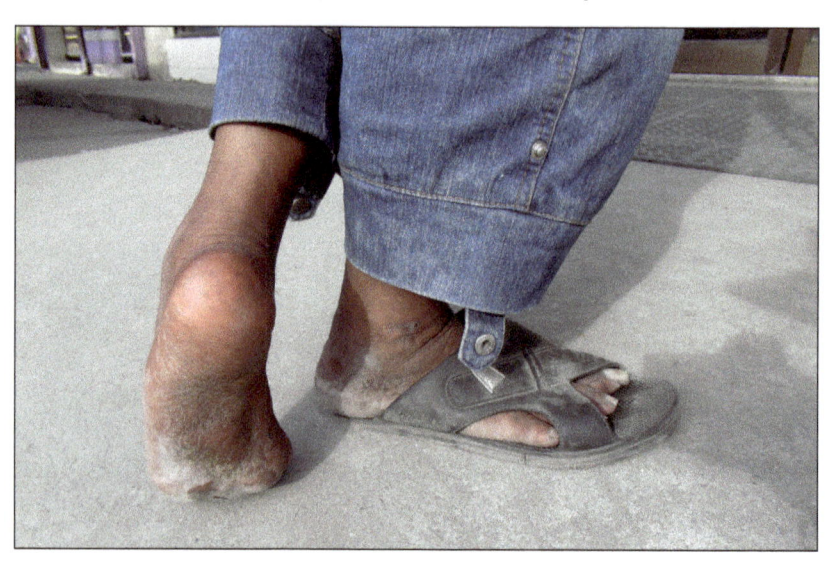

Posterior (Back) View Left Foot Equinovarus

Source: https://commons.wikimedia.org/wiki/File:Clubfoot_beggar_with_cane_04.jpg

In this example, the posture of the thigh, leg, and foot is known as an extension synergy pattern. Muscles in the front of the thigh (quadriceps group) keeps the knee straight. Muscles of the calf cause the foot to point straight down (gastrocnemius and soleus, also known as triceps surae) or down and rotated in (tibialis posterior).

Posterior (Back) View Triceps Surae

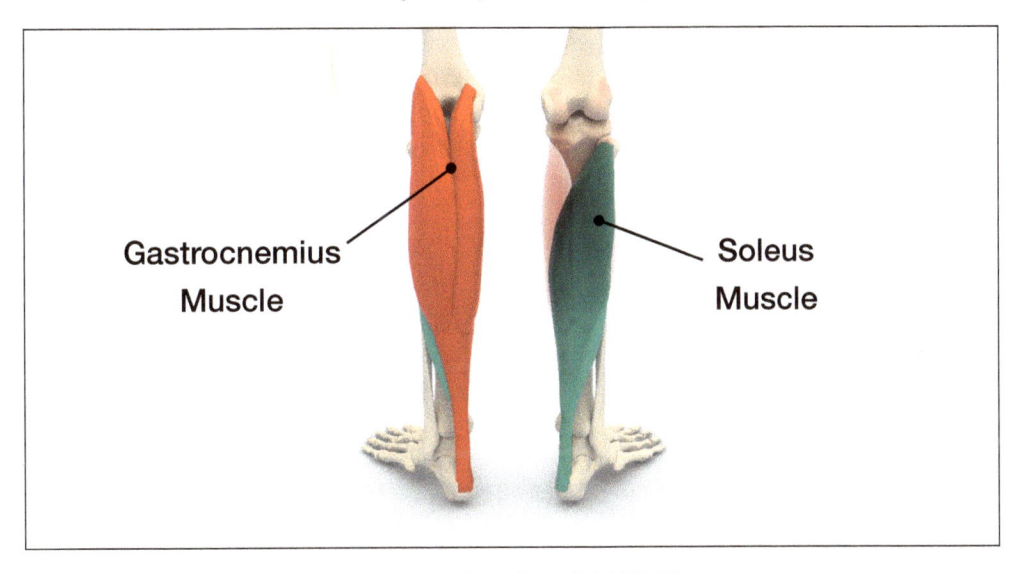

Source: https://commons.wikimedia.org/wiki/File:Triceps_surae.svg

Posterior (Back) View Tibialis Posterior

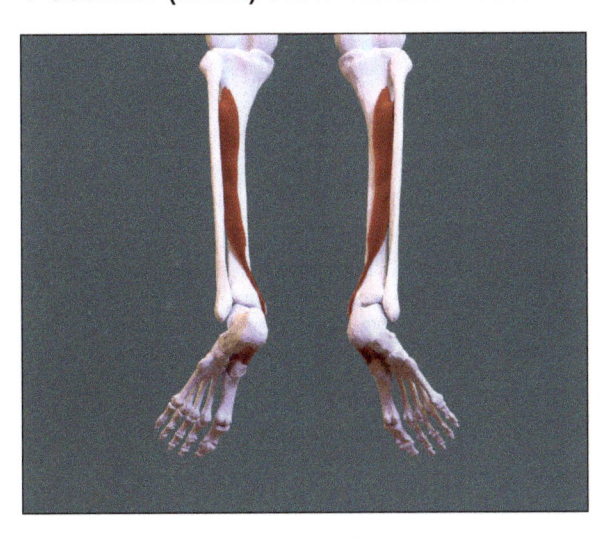

Source: https://commons.wikimedia.org/wiki/File:Inferior_view_of_tibialis_posterior_muscle_-_posterior.png

The ankle position tends to be stiff. A contracture or hardening of the Achilles tendon (heel cord) in the back of the ankle or the tibialis posterior tendon causes the ankle to become immobile, often requiring surgical intervention.

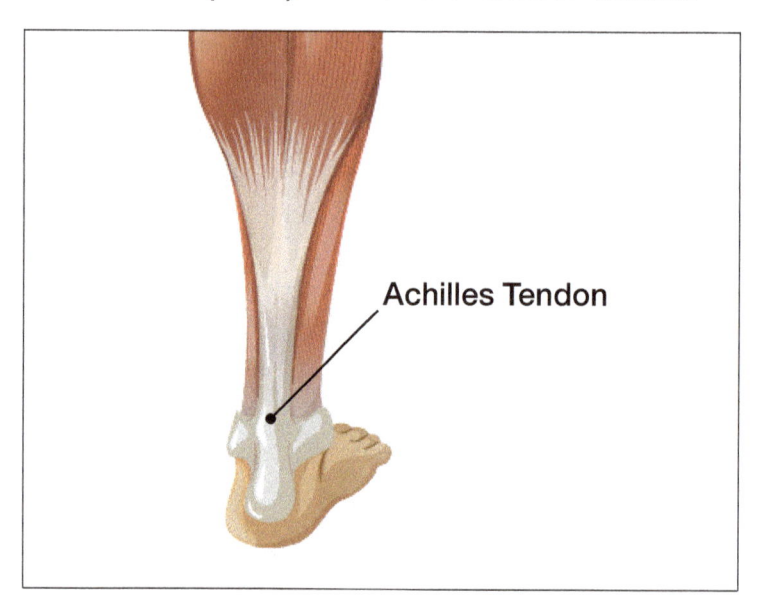

Posterior (Back) View of the Achilles Tendon

Achilles Tendon

Plantarflexed Foot Due to Contracture of the Achilles Tendon

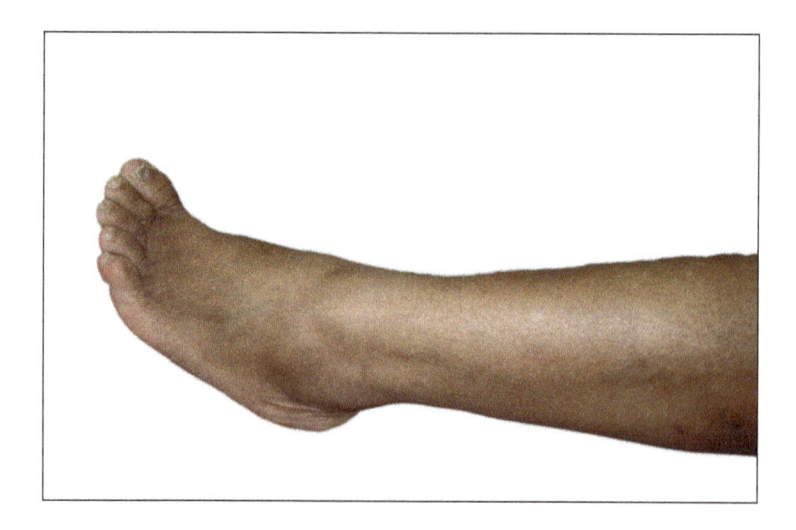

If there is some movement of the foot moving up, but it is difficult and the Achilles tendon is stiff, then a series of casts can be applied to slowly stretch the Achilles tendon so the foot can move up.

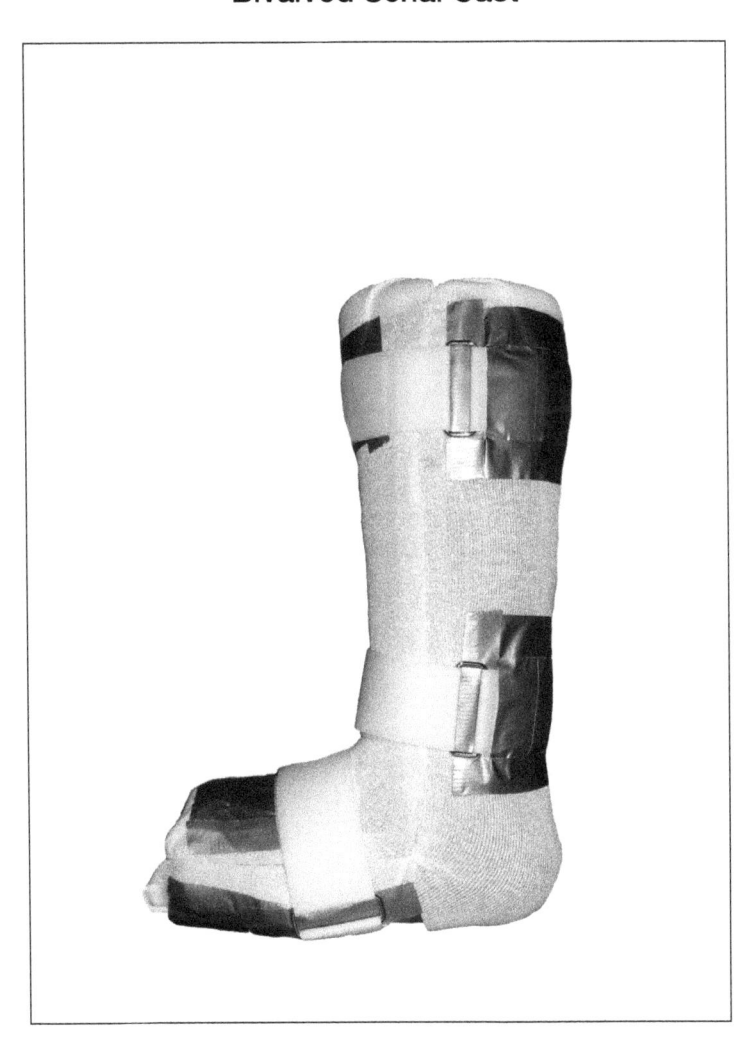

Bivalved Serial Cast

CHAPTER 3

What Is An AFO?

An ankle foot orthosis or AFO is a type of brace which is applied to the leg and foot for support when the muscles are weak or has abnormal muscle tone (tension) from a brain injury such as a stroke.[28] It is primarily to keep the foot from pointing down or "dropping."

The AFO has three basic parts:

1. A footplate that touches the bottom and side of the foot

2. A shaft that surrounds portions of the back and sides of the leg

3. Straps to secure the brace to the leg, ankle, and foot

The AFO can be solid at the ankle or hinged making it possible for the footplate or the shaft to move. The trimlines or edges of the AFO that covers the leg, ankle, and foot vary depending on muscle weakness, muscle tone (tension), and bone stability.

AFO Anterior (Front) View

- Shaft
- Strap
- Footplate

Hinged AFO Lateral (Side) View

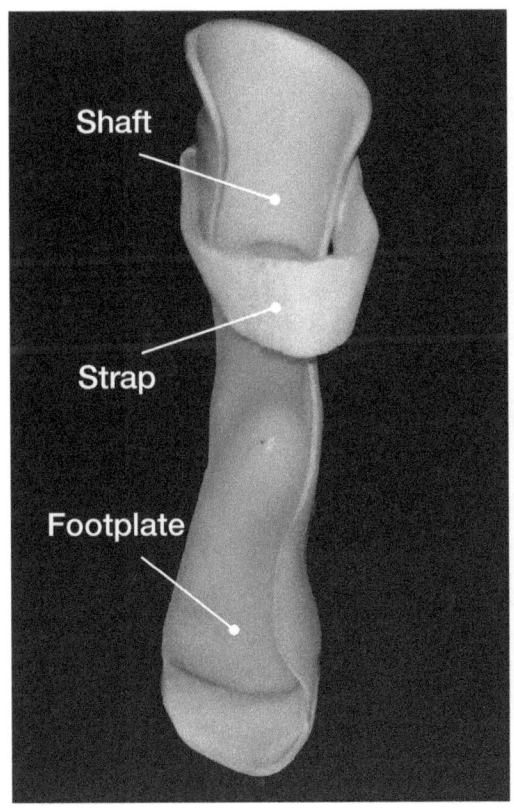

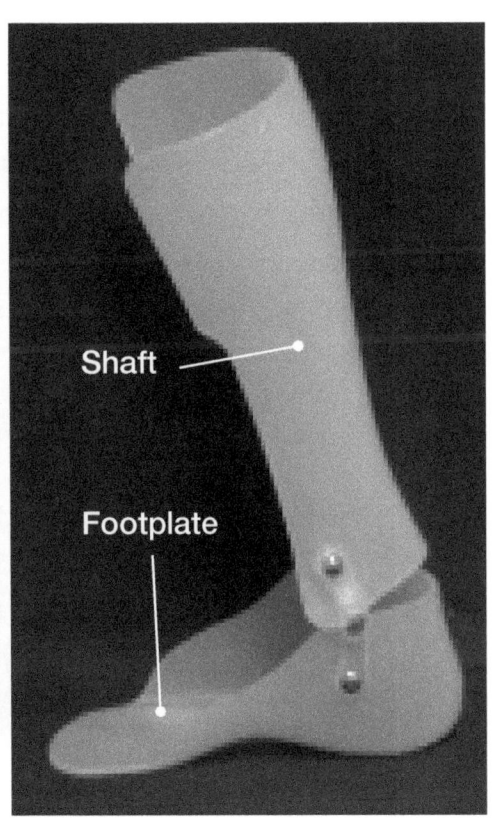

- Shaft
- Footplate

CHAPTER 4

Why Do I Need An AFO?

The purpose of the AFO is to hold the foot up when the leg is in the air, so you do not trip on or over the foot. The AFO stabilizes the foot when it is on the ground, but it often restricts the leg from moving forward during walking, standing up or sitting down. The leg moving forward is a natural part of movement during walking, standing up or sitting down. It is not necessary to restrict the leg movement forward during walking, standing up or sitting down if the muscles that control the foot are weak, floppy or stiff.

Lateral (Outside) View of Left Leg at Terminal Stance

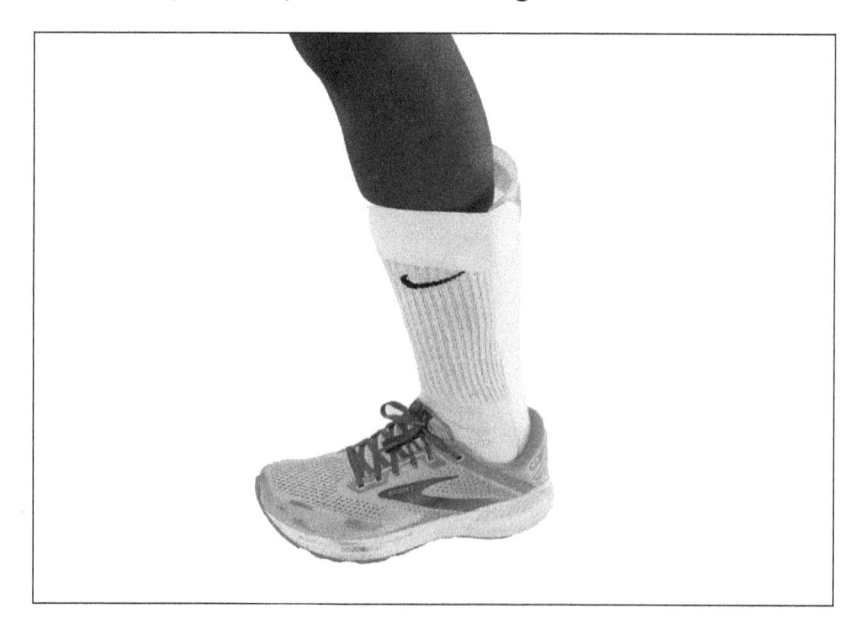

Lateral (Outside) View
Right Leg Sit to Stand

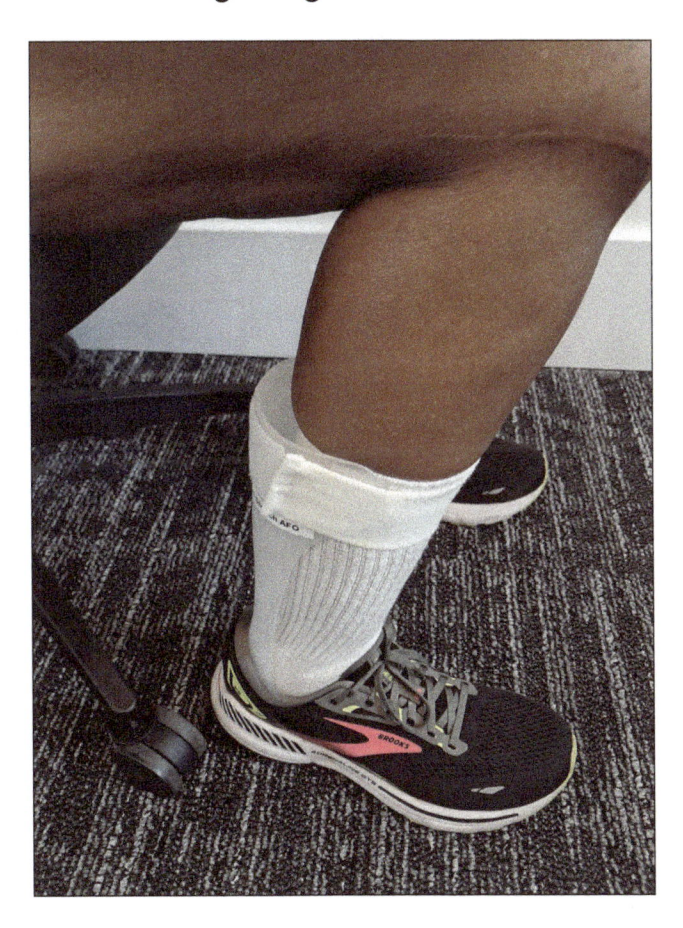

CHAPTER 5

What Should My Physical Therapist (PT) Do?

The PT should conduct a thorough examination to tell the orthotist about problems you have because of the stroke or brain injury. This information assures recommendations for the best AFO. Once made to properly fit your foot and shoe, the AFO may improve your walking and engaging in daily home, work or leisure activities.

Physical Therapy Examination Components[29]

- **Postural observation:** Compare foot positions in a weightbearing (WB) activity (standing and sitting with feet on floor or surface) and a non-weightbearing (NWB) activity (sitting with feet dangling)

- **Abnormal foot appearance and subsequent compensations:** Problems from the stroke or brain injury (for example, weakness and muscle stiffness) may cause the foot to:

    a. be flat - no arches (pronation) or

    b. have an abnormally high arch on the inside of the foot (supination) or

    c. have positioning differences between the hindfoot (heel), midfoot (middle), and forefoot (distal part of the foot including toes).

- Range of motion (joint flexibility):

    a. Measured with the foot not on the floor or surface (non-weightbearing) with knee straight and bent; usually laying on back (best) or sitting in a chair

    b. Measured with the foot on the floor or surface (weightbearing) with knee straight and bent; standing position is best

- **Strength and Voluntary Control:** Isolated movement of one muscle or a group of muscles working together to move a body part
- **Pathological Reflexes:** Abnormal movement of the foot caused by stimulation to the bottom of the foot when it is in weightbearing on the floor, ground or a surface; this abnormal movement can lead to unsafe walking
- **Spasticity:** The muscle is stretched at a fast speed resulting in movement of the body part in the opposite direction of the stretch; the movement looks like a clasp-knife closing, thus called a clasp-knife response
- **Tone:** Muscle tension that is developed when a body part is moved to lengthen the muscle from its shortest position; the tension or tone is characterized as flaccid (floppy), hypotonia (low tone) or hypertonia (high tone – stiff or rigid)
- **Sensation:** Measuring your ability to feel the position of a joint (proprioception), measuring your ability to copy the movement direction of multiple joints (kinesthesia), and measuring the ability to feel a plastic wire on your skin (monofilament testing)
- **Balance:** Static (sitting and standing still) or dynamic (moving while sitting or standing) using a test based on type and location of the stroke or brain injury
- **Edema (swelling):** Location, type, when is there the most or least amount of swelling, and what increases or decreases the swelling

- **Pain:** Location, intensity, description, and what relieves or intensifies the pain
- **Vision:** Assessing visual field cut or hemianopsia which is seeing half of the environment out of both eyes versus visual neglect which is detecting your ability to process and interact with what is seen in the environment
- **Functional Mobility Assessment:** Assessing getting in and out of bed, sit to stand (STS) and falls analysis (getting down to and up from floor) but can also include things important to you like getting in and out of a car
- **Walking:** Assessing speed (how fast you walk) and quality (what your walking looks like)
- **Personal Items:** Things you use on or with your body during the day like a purse, backpack, briefcase, and or umbrella
- **Level of function:**

    a. **Prior:** What you use to do in terms of daily activities

    b. **Current:** What you are doing now in terms of daily activities after the stroke or brain injury

- **Goals:** Short-term while in therapy and long-term which is after therapy is complete
- **Treatment:** Exercises and or therapeutic activities related to your goals with and without the AFO; furthermore, the PT should measure improvement in your leg and foot function and tell the orthotist this information so the AFO can be modified

CHAPTER 6

What Should I Ask My PT?

1. What is your experience in making recommendations for AFOs?

2. Will you be present at the initial meeting with the orthotist?

3. What information do you need from me to write a letter of medical necessity so that the insurance will pay for the AFO?

    NOTE: Make sure you know insurance coverage and out of pocket costs amongst other things.

4. What information will be provided to the orthotist from the physical therapy examination?

5. How will this information be communicated? For example, written documentation, pictures, and or videos

6. What determines the type of AFO I will get?

7. What activities will be done without the AFO to allow potential recovery of problems like muscle strength or range of motion and or efficient and effective improvement of functional recovery like sit to stand (STS) or walking on different surfaces?

8. What activities will be done with the AFO to promote efficient, effective, and meaningful functional recovery such as walking safely and faster, preventing

falls, and negotiating stairs and uneven surfaces even though strength or range of motion may not improve?

NOTE: Number seven and eight should have some distinct lists of activities, not all of the same activities.

CHAPTER 7

What Should My Orthotist Do?

Remember the orthotist gets reimbursed a fixed amount to make an AFO. The time spent with you and the PT is critical for the initial fabrication process and the initial and follow-up fitting sessions. Therefore, be respectful of everyone's time and come with your comments and questions ready. The orthotist should first collaborate with you and the PT.

The process of getting an AFO should include:

1. a consultation among the orthotist, PT, and you.

2. a pre-casting or scanning (process using equipment to take a picture or video of the leg and foot) assessment which the orthotist does taking into consideration the examination information provided by the PT.

3. recommending the best AFO whether it is custom or prefabricated (off-the-shelf).

4. the casting procedure if a custom AFO is recommended.

5. an initial fitting session with or without the PT, and

6. any follow-up sessions as needed to change the AFO based on initial problems and or improvement in those problems such as weakness, range of motion, muscle tone (tension), and or spasticity (clasp-knife movement of the

distal body segment, usually the foot).

The orthotist is the expert on materials to make the AFO and the properties of those materials like stiffness, wear, and tear. The orthotist should recommend the best AFO based on material properties and how the AFO should fit and function whether it is prefabricated or custom.

Most importantly, the AFO should accommodate social determinants of health[1] (education access and quality, economic stability, health care access and quality, neighborhood and built environment, and social and community context [going out and socializing with people]) that is reflective of your lifestyle. For example, your preference for shoes, clothing or the circumstances of your daily activities be it work or leisure.

Last, inform the orthotist if you have someone present to help you put on and take off the AFO and the shoe. If no one is available, demonstrate to the orthotist how you put on and take off your shoe, preferably, the one you want to wear with the AFO.

CHAPTER 8

What Should I Ask My Orthotist?

1. Are you willing to consult with a PT regarding my baseline function, current level of function, and potential for improved walking?

2. What is the added cost to change the AFO to accommodate my specific problems (for example, weakness and muscle stiffness), shoe and clothing preference, and values (for example, flesh tone color material)?

3. What is the process of making the AFO to fit into one of my regularly worn shoes?

    NOTE:

    a. Ankle range of motion measurements in various positions should provide clues whether you should wear a flat or a wedge heel shoe.

    b. Bring the pair of shoes you previously wore the most and or want to wear with the AFO.

4. What is the process for modifications over time? For example, muscles on the side of my leg and foot get stronger requiring a less obtrusive AFO.

5. What is the associated cost for modifications?

6. Do you make the AFO locally at your facility or send it out to a vendor?

7. If sent out to be made, to whom and where is this vendor located?

> **NOTE:** Do your research to verify the vendor's experience with making custom ordered AFOs and verify customer satisfaction or complaints.

8. Is this vendor open to fabricating an AFO specific for my needs?

9. How will information, such as written documentation, pictures, and or videos, be communicated about my problems (for example, weakness and muscle stiffness) and value preferences regarding the AFO?

10. What does the insole of my shoe say about my normal weightbearing foot pattern prior to the stroke or brain injury?

11. How might the footplate of the AFO be structured to accommodate what is normal versus what may have changed due to the stroke or brain injury?

12. What does the wear pattern on the exterior portions of my shoe say about my normal weightbearing foot pattern prior to the stroke from when my foot first touches the floor, ground or any surface until the last portion of my foot leaves the floor, ground or any surface?

13. How might this information be used to change the AFO and still provide the function needed to accommodate my problems (for example, weakness and muscle stiffness)?

14. How might this information be used to suggest the best shoe for me that will accommodate the AFO?

15. Furthermore, what are the characteristics of the shoe that would best accommodate the AFO?

    a. Flat or wedge sole

    b. Pointed or round toe box

    c. Forefoot flat or curved up

    d. Extra depth of the toe box

    e. Heel shape and depth

    f. Shoelaces, Velcro® or zipper to secure the shoe and the location

    g. Shoe material

16. What are the characteristics of the AFO that I need based on my problems (for example, weakness and muscle stiffness) and why?

17. Is there another choice besides using rigid Velcro® straps with a metal link rectangular in shape at the top of the AFO or across the ankle or foot?

    a. Rigid straps prevent the leg from moving forward at the knee joint and at the ankle joint, the latter impacting movement at the midfoot.

    b. The body weight is unable to shift efficiently and effectively from behind to in front of the body, especially when a rigid calf and or ankle/foot strap is used on a custom made solid AFO.

    c. An elastic strap that can control leg movement based on muscle sensorimotor function is a better option; more elasticity for stronger muscles and less elasticity for weaker muscles.

18. What is the wearing schedule to get use to my AFO?

19. What are some signs to look for if the AFO is not fitting right?

20. What are some signs to look for if the AFO is not functioning properly (for example, hold my foot up when my leg is up in the air or does not allow my leg to come forward when my foot is on the floor, ground or a surface) when I stand up, walk or sit down?

21. What type of socks or compression garment can I wear with the AFO?

22. What should I do if my leg, ankle, and or foot swells?

    NOTE: The time of day, amount of swelling, and classification of swelling (Grades 1-4 which explains the time it takes for fluid to settle back in place once displaced) should be a part of physical therapy examination information given to the orthotist.

23. What should I do to get rid of the odor from sweating/perspiration?

24. How do I keep the AFO clean?

25. When can I get another AFO per insurance guidelines?

    NOTE: Be specific for your insurance company. Most follow Medicare rules and guidelines.

CHAPTER 9

What To Expect When I Get the AFO: Fit & Function

If the leg and foot is low tone or floppy, the AFO should:

1. hold the foot parallel to the floor or the ground and or surface that is level when the leg is up in the air (swing phase).

2. not stop the leg from moving forward when your foot is on a level surface such as the floor or the ground while walking nor during standing up or sitting down.

3. allow you to roll over your toes and allow the knee to bend right before the foot leaves the ground if the toeplate (part of the AFO under the toes) extends to the end of the toes. Therefore, the toeplate should be flexible and not necessarily flat but have a slight arch from the little (fifth) toe to the big (first) toe.

4. accommodate your natural foot position if you are a natural pronator (foot flat) or supinator (high arch).

5. be made to accommodate stronger versus weaker muscles. For example, if your muscles are strong that control the foot turning in or out, the shaft trimlines do not have to come in front of the malleoli (protruding bony parts of the ankle).

6. accommodate the protruding bony parts of the leg, ankle, and foot with little to no chafing/rubbing when the leg moves forward and or backwards, particularly when your foot is on a level surface like the floor or the ground.

7. be made to the shape of your foot especially so that with it on, your foot is comfortable in the shoe. There may have to be some special accommodations:

    a. If the ankle is inflexible (lacks range of motion) and the foot is pointed down, a wedge may be added to the outside heel of the AFO to take up space between the heel and the floor or inner sole of the shoe. When this is done, the lower extremity appears longer, and the opposite shoe may have to be changed to account for the length difference. The opposite shoe will have external layers added to the external sole or a recommendation for both shoes to have a built in wedged sole to accommodate the foot pointed down.

Posterior (Back) View of AFO Wedge

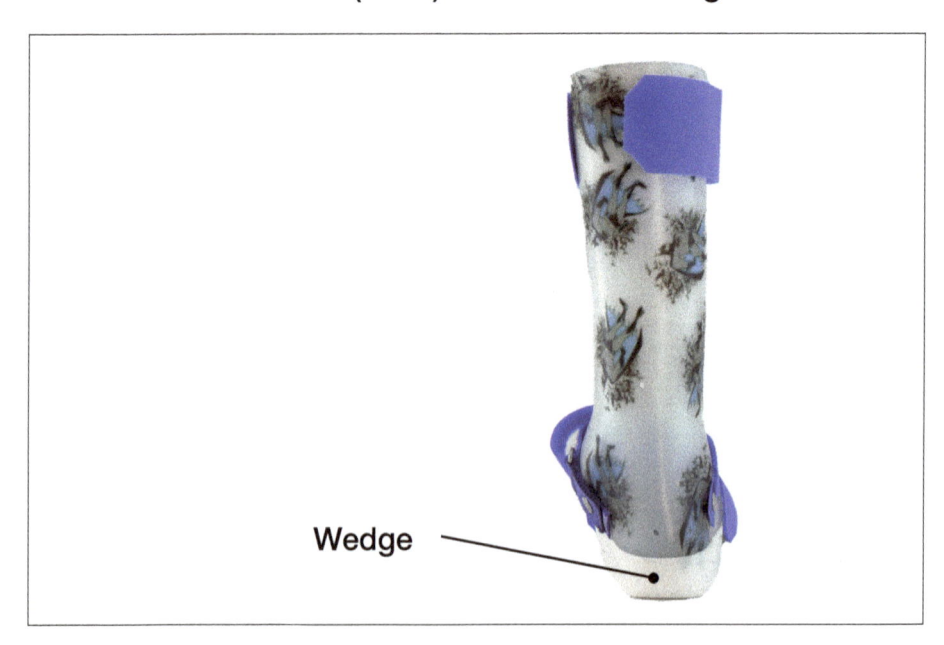

Wedge

b. Sometimes the AFO is purposely set in plantarflexion (foot pointed down) to raise the heel causing the knee to bend, thus preventing the knee from being behind the hip and ankle. This does not always work because ankle joint range of motion loss may result in ankle contracture (no movement) and the leg is unable to move forward resulting in an abnormal position in which the knee is behind the ankle (hyperextension).

Ankle range of motion loss is often a result of:

- increased muscle tone/tension (increase stiffness or rigidity) in the calf muscles and the anterior thigh muscles,

- Achilles tendon (heel cord) stiffness or contracture (no flexibility), and or

- the tibialis anterior and fibularis longus muscles are not strong enough to pull the foot up.

CHAPTER 10

Physical Therapy Pearls From Career Experiences

- ☑ Individuals with stroke who have visual neglect tend to have a poor functional outcome in mobility because they are not visually interacting with or processing information they see in the environment, often resulting in falls.

- ☑ Individuals with stroke who have hemianopsia, a visual field cut, tend to have a poor functional outcome in mobility if they *do not* learn to scan the environment or use prism glasses, often resulting in running into objects or falls because they only see items in one half of the environment.

- ☑ Individuals with stroke with an extensor synergy pattern (knee straight and foot pointed down) tend to be better walkers than those with a flexor synergy pattern (hip and knee bent and foot pointed up), because the latter group cannot keep their foot on the floor, ground or any surface for stance phase.

- ☑ Individuals with stroke who exercised regularly before the stroke or brain injury tend to have better functional mobility with activities that include moving in bed, sit to stand and vice versa, transfers (for example, moving from the wheelchair to and from the bed), and walking on level and unlevel surfaces (ramps/inclines and stairs).

- ☑ Despite having to wear an AFO for the long-term, which demonstrates weakness in the foot, you should not let that deter you from exercising. Exercising at any level or engaging in physical activity after stroke prevents the likelihood of having a second stroke. Overall, exercise and or physical activity is good for your health.

- ☑ Be prepared to buy two pairs of shoes especially if you have narrow or shorter feet. An extra-long and wide shoe can make steps on your leg not affected by the stroke or brain injury more apt to tripping, causing a potential fall.

- ☑ Do as many exercises as possible safely without the AFO to maintain and increase joint range of motion (flexibility) and or strength. Tell your PT and orthotist if you have a gain or loss in range of motion or strength so that the AFO can be modified to accommodate those changes.

- ☑ Communicate your hopes and fears so that they can be addressed. Be open to what sounds positive and perceived as negative. For everything that may sound negative, there is a solution that can be done to turn it into a positive so that you can safely function at some level of independence.

Afterward

I know this was a lot of detailed information. I wrote this book to prepare anyone dealing with the aftereffects of a stroke for what should be expected when having an AFO made. You as an individual with stroke or any neurologic diagnosis, a caregiver, an examining physical therapist or a treating physical therapy practitioner, and an orthotist or pedorthist should be better at asking and answering questions. I hope this book serves as a guide to bring everyone together to communicate the needs and wants of the individual with stroke. As an individual with stroke or any person with a neurologic diagnosis, I hope you and your caregiver are equipped and empowered to win at health. This resource guide should set the agenda on how an AFO can be made for you and what you want to do. I encourage you and or your caregiver to be an advocate for your health. If exercise is medicine and walking is exercise, then it all starts with an AFO. Happy walking, but more importantly, happy living!

References

1. Healthy People 2030, U.S. Department of Health and Human Services, Office of Disease Prevention and Health Promotion. Retrieved March 17, 2023, from https://health.gov/healthypeople/objectives-and-data/social-determinants-health

2. Neumann DA. Chapter 13: Knee. In Neumann DA, ed. *Kinesiology of the Musculoskeletal System: Foundations for Rehabilitation*. 2nd ed. Mosby/Elsevier; 2010:520-572.

3. Neumann DA. Chapter 14: Ankle and foot. In Neumann DA, ed. *Kinesiology of the Musculoskeletal System: Foundations for Rehabilitation*. 2nd ed. Mosby/Elsevier; 2010:573-626.

4. Babu D, Bordoni B. Anatomy, Bony Pelvis and Lower Limb, Medial Longitudinal Arch of the Foot. [Updated 2022 Nov 11]. In: StatPearls [Internet]. Treasure Island (FL): StatPearls Publishing; 2022 Jan-. Available from: https://www.ncbi.nlm.nih.gov/books/NBK562289/

5. Stills M. Thermoformed ankle-foot orthoses. *Orthot Prosthet*. 1975;29(4):41-51.

6. Fergus A, Fell DW, Wellons RT. Chapter 9: Examination of balance and equilibrium. In Fell DW, Lunnen KY, Rauk RP, eds. *Lifespan Neurorehabilitation: A Patient-Centered Approach from Examination to Interventions and Outcomes*. F. A. Davis Company; 2018:238-280.

7. Neumann DA. Chapter 15: Kinesiology of walking. In Neumann DA, ed. *Kinesiology of the Musculoskeletal System: Foundations for Rehabilitation*. 2nd ed. Mosby/Elsevier; 2010:627-681.

8. Simpkins SD, Zipp GP, Fell DW. Chapter 37: Functional activity intervention in upright mobility. In Fell DW, Lunnen KY, Rauk RP, eds. *Lifespan Neurorehabilitation: A Patient-Centered Approach from Examination to Interventions and Outcomes*. F. A. Davis Company; 2018:1132-1168.

9. Pathokinesiology Service & the Physical Therapy Department. *Observational Gait Analysis*. 4th ed. Rancho Los Amigos National Rehabilitation Center, Downey, CA: Los Amigos Research and Educational Institute; 2001.

10. Fell DW. Chapter 5: Examination and evaluation of sensory systems. In Fell DW, Lunnen KY, Rauk RP, eds. *Lifespan Neurorehabilitation: A Patient-Centered Approach from Examination to Interventions and Outcomes*. F. A. Davis Company; 2018:115-142.

11. Neumann DA. Chapter 1: Getting started. In Neumann DA, ed. *Kinesiology of the Musculoskeletal System: Foundations for Rehabilitation*. 2nd ed. Mosby/Elsevier; 2010:1-27.

12. Fell DW. Chapter 15: General approaches to neurological rehabilitation. In Fell DW, Lunnen KY, Rauk RP, eds. *Lifespan Neurorehabilitation: A Patient-Centered Approach from Examination to Interventions and Outcomes*. F. A. Davis Company; 2018:490-523.

13. Rauk RP, Dunfee H. Chapter 18: Intervention for flaccidity and hypotonia: spastic and rigid. In Fell DW, Lunnen KY, Rauk RP, eds. *Lifespan Neurorehabilitation: A Patient-Centered Approach from Examination to Interventions and Outcomes*. F. A. Davis Company; 2018:605-629.

14. O'Shea RK, White L, Fell DW. Chapter 19: Intervention related to hypertonia: spastic and rigid. In Fell DW, Lunnen KY, Rauk RP, eds. *Lifespan Neuroreha-

bilitation: A Patient-Centered Approach from Examination to Interventions and Outcomes*. F. A. Davis Company; 2018:630-648.

15. Duncan W. Tonic reflexes of the foot. *J Bone Joint Surg*.1960; 42:859-868.

16. Fell DW. Chapter 6: Examination and evaluation in neuromuscular disorders. In Fell DW, Lunnen KY, Rauk RP, eds. *Lifespan Neurorehabilitation: A Patient-Centered Approach from Examination to Interventions and Outcomes*. F. A. Davis Company; 2018:143-190.

17. Levin MF, Kleim JA, Wolf SL. What do motor "recovery" and "compensation" mean in patients following stroke? *Neurorehabil Neural Repair*. 2009;23(4):313-319. doi:10.1177/1545968308328727

18. O'Dell MW, Lin CC, Harrison V. Stroke rehabilitation: strategies to enhance motor recovery. *Annu Rev Med*. 2009;60:55-68.doi:10.1146/annurev.med.60.042707.104248

19. Watson L. Shoe terminology: Anatomy of a shoe. Hoodmwr.com. Updated June 16, 2022. Accessed February 27, 2023. https://www.hoodmwr.com/anatomy-of-the-shoe/

20. Dupere K. The anatomy of a sneaker explained: Everything you need to know about the parts of your shoes & how they work. Footwearnews.com. January 25, 2022. Accessed February 27, 2023. https://footwearnews.com/feature/parts-of-sneakers-1203233336/

21. Lundy-Ekman L. Chapter 14: Motor system: motor tracts. In Lundy-Ekman L, ed. *Neuroscience, Fundamentals for Rehabilitation*. 5th ed. Saunders Elsevier; 2018:258-289.

22. Harro CC, Wilcox KC. Chapter 22: Interventions for weakness in neuromotor disorders. In Fell DW, Lunnen KY, Rauk RP, eds. *Lifespan Neurorehabilitation: A Patient-Centered Approach from Examination to Interventions and Outcomes*. F. A. Davis Company; 2018:725-755.

23. Park BS, Kim MY, Lee LK et al. The effects of a progressive resistance training program on walking ability in patients after stroke. *J Phys Ther Sci*. 2015;27(9):2837-2840.

24. Lundy-Ekman L, Peterson C. Chapter 13: Motor system: motor neurons and spinal motor function. In Lundy-Ekman L, ed. *Neuroscience, Fundamentals for Rehabilitation*. 5th ed. Saunders Elsevier; 2018:241-257.

25. Fell DW. Chapter 7: Examination and evaluation of cranial nerves. In Fell DW, Lunnen KY, Rauk RP, eds. *Lifespan Neurorehabilitation: A Patient-Centered Approach from Examination to Interventions and Outcomes*. F. A. Davis Company; 2018:191-209.

26. Warren M. *Brain Injury Visual Assessment Battery for Adults: Test Manual*. Birmingham, AL: VisAbilities Rehab Services, Inc.;1988:4-43, Ref 2.

27. Garcia JM, Cardell B, Fell DW, Champley J. Chapter 31: Overcoming challenges of impaired perception, cognition, and communication (aphasia or dysarthria). In Fell DW, Lunnen KY, Rauk RP, eds. *Lifespan Neurorehabilitation: A Patient-Centered Approach from Examination to Interventions and Outcomes*. F. A. Davis Company; 2018:978-994.

28. Lovegreen W, Pai AB. Chapter 32: Orthoses for the muscle diseased patient. In Webster JB, Murphy DP, eds. *Atlas of Orthoses and Assistive Devices*. 5th ed. Elsevier; 2019:332-336.e1.

29. Alazzawi S, Sukeik M, King D, Vemulapalli K. Foot and ankle history and clinical examination: A guide to everyday practice. *World Journal of Orthopedics*. 2017;8(1):21-29. doi:10.5312/wjo.v8.i1.21.

Publications

Brown JV, Suhr J. Quantifying AFO use, fit & function via outcome measures by physical therapists. *IJAHSP*. In press.

Brown JV, Best S, Suhr J. Ankle Foot Orthoses: The Impact of Appearance, Function, and Fit in Individuals with Stroke. *Lower Extremity Review*. 2021;13(11):39-50. Available at: https://lermagazine.com/cover_story/ankle-foot-orthoses-the-impact-of-appearance-function-and-fit-in-individuals-with-stroke

Brown JV, Cotton J, Best S, Suhr JA. Communicating key features of an ankle foot orthosis from a patient's perspective: a case study. *J NSAH*. 2020; 17(1):6-20.

Peer Reviewed Scientific and Professional Presentations

Brown JV. Individuals with stroke speak about AFOs. We need team talk for a better walk. Paper presented at: Ohio Chapter of the American Academy of Orthotists and Prosthetists 2021 Annual Conference. March 13, 2021; OH

Brown JV. Custom ankle foot orthosis fabrication using 3-D printing. Panel discussion accepted but not presented at: Ohio Physical Therapy Association 2018 Annual Conference. April 13, 2018; Columbus, OH.

Brown JV. The physical therapist's role in assessment for AFOs: A 3-D point of view. Accepted but not presented at: Ohio Physical Therapy Association 2018 Annual Conference. April 13, 2018; Columbus, OH.

Brown JV. Photovoice and videovoice: The art of communicating user preferences for solid ankle foot orthosis post stroke. Poster presented at: American Physical Therapy Association 2018 Combined Sections Meeting. February 24, 2018; New Orleans, LA

About the Author

Jennifaye V. Brown is a PhD-trained physical therapist who has been board certified as a neurologic clinical specialist by the American Board of Physical Therapy Specialties of the American Physical Therapy Association (APTA) for four 10-year terms. She is a neurodevelopmental treatment (NDT)-trained therapist with six additional courses taken after the NDT (Bobath) Three Week Course on Treatment of Adult Hemiplegia. While teaching students in various healthcare settings as an Advanced Credentialed Clinical Instructor by the Clinical Instructor Education Board of the APTA, Dr. Brown taught in the neuromuscular curriculum in physical therapy and physical therapy assistant programs and now teaches continuing education courses on adult neurologic examination and treatment intervention for acquired brain injury, particularly stroke. Dr. Brown's research agenda explored the 1) perceptions and opinions of individuals with stroke regarding their experiences with AFO fabrication, modification, and maintenance and how the AFO impacts walking and participation in life roles and 2) use of tests or outcome measures by physical therapists to determine AFO fit, function, and use.

Dr. Brown currently resides in Charleston, South Carolina. As the owner of jvb physical therapy services llc, she values collaborating and consulting with individuals with brain injury (particularly stroke), caregivers, physical therapy practitioners, and orthotists (people who specialize in making an AFO) to make the best AFO for fit and function based on a comprehensive examination. She is a Certified Aging in Place Specialist who is experienced in accessibility home design allowing individuals with all types of brain injuries to safely age in place.

Dr. Brown has made recommendations to adapt homes of individuals with chronic impairments whose goal was to improve their mobility resulting in 90% able to safely walk, exercise, and engage in physical activities with a custom AFO that she designed. As a certified personal trainer, Dr. Brown is an exercise enthusiast and enjoys teaching aquatic fitness classes. Dr. Brown is a member of the APTA, Neurology Section of the APTA, SC Chapter of the APTA, Athletics & Fitness Association of America, and a graduate of the prestigious APTA Fellowship in Education Leadership.

Certifications

- Certified Neurologic Clinical Specialist for four 10-year terms by the American Board of Physical Therapy Specialties, American Physical Therapy Association
- Certified Aging in Place Specialist, National Association of Home Builders
- Certified Personal Trainer, Athletics & Fitness Association of America

---

"Dr. Brown is a very experienced neuro specialist physical therapist with a vast knowledge base of many topics in neurology but has chosen one here to help those survivors of stroke/brain injury to have improved mobility through the use of an ankle-foot-orthosis (AFO). Dr. Brown has provided a wonderful resource for those person(s) who have had a stroke/brain injury, or any neurologic disorder with resultant lower leg impairments that have had problems with falls, balance and overall limited mobility that could benefit from the use of an AFO. The resource booklet that she has written is thorough and provides a complete education for those persons to be their own advocate with interest in an AFO device that could potentially improve their home and community involvement. The resource provides the why, what, with who, how to achieve obtaining an AFO. The resource provides a thorough understanding of the need and advantages of the use of an AFO. This is a highly recommended resource for those interested in improving their mobility due to foot drop, spasticity, and or weakness in the lower limb from their neurologic injury."

Terri Kazanjian, MSPT
Former Manager of the Acquired Brain Injury Unit, Shepherd Center, Atlanta, GA

AFOs Designed by Dr. Jennifaye V. Brown

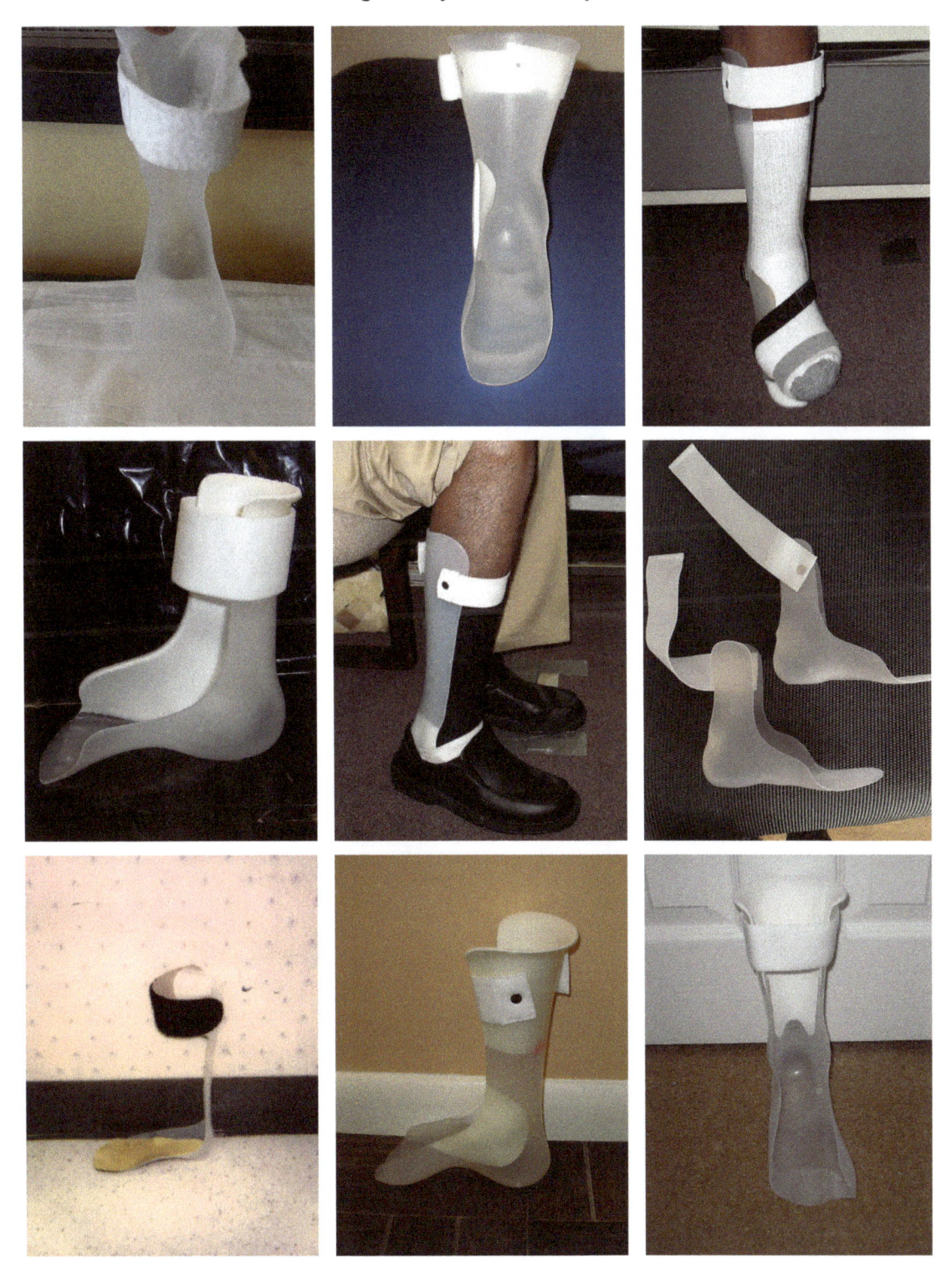